THE SERGEANT'S FITNESS AND NUTRITION PROGRAM

Photographs by David Brooks

A Fireside Book   Published by Simon & Schuster

BOOT CAMP

BE ALL YOU USED TO BE

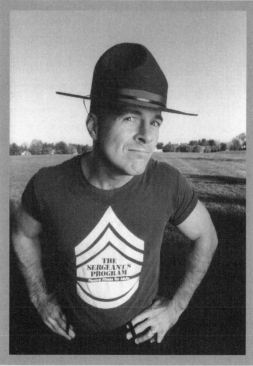

Patrick "The Sarge" Avon and Maryann Karinch

FIRESIDE
Rockefeller Center
1230 Avenue of the Americas
New York, NY 10020

FIRESIDE and colophon are registered trademarks
of Simon & Schuster Inc.

Designed by Bonni Leon-Berman

Manufactured in the United States of America

1 3 5 7 9 10 8 6 4 2

Library of Congress Cataloging-in-Publication Data

Avon, Patrick.
Boot camp : be all you used to be : the sergeant's fitness and
nutrition program / Patrick Avon and Maryann Karinch ; photographs
by David Brooks.
p. cm.
"A Fireside book."
Includes index.
1. Physical fitness—Popular works. 2. Reducing exercises—
Popular works. 3. Reducing diets—Popular works. 4. Nutrition—
Popular works. I. Karinch, Maryann. II. Title.
RA781.A94 1999
613.7—dc21   98-37013 CIP
ISBN 0-684-84899-6

CONTENTS

ACKNOWLEDGMENTS

We jointly thank our loving partners at home, Bridgit Avon and James McCormick, for their patience and insights, as well as Isaac Hunter Avon, who was smart enough to come into this world after we had completed the first draft. Laura Belt and Lisa Swayne of Adler & Robin Books brought us together and supported our work in every way. Our gifted editor, Sarah Baker, helped us stay on track. Photographer David Brooks put heart, as well as talent, into this project. Exercise Physiologist Mark Occhipinti, President of American Fitness Professionals and Associates, contributed valuable expertise. Our program staff made our work together even more fun and productive—Rob Jardeleza, Abby Bloomenstock, Connie Kellogg, Fred "The Hammer" Foster, Ahmad "Ashey Knees" Coston, Lawrence Witner, Patrick "Major" Riley, Brian Sulc, Peter Lohrey, Stew Smith, Kirk Herrick, Bob "BullDog" Zimmermann, Mary Forté, Tim Seals, Steve Day, Donna Garnett, Chuck "Six-ups" Dyson, Brett Schleuter, Joe Loza, Bill "Big Butt" Isola, Dimitri Louis, Kabba Jones, Bill Hoss, Jason Beakes, Ben Braman, Jason Colosky, Karen Baines, Brent Harder, Margo Bailey, and all other instructors and staff from the past. All past and present clients have made Boot Camp and this book strong and fun; special thanks to those who let us include their faces, bodies, and stories in this book—Andy Betterman, Charles Kim, Steve Pugliese, Gerald Zapol, Jeff Witte, Frank Bell, Charles Harmel, Maurice Werner, Trish Hamilton, Brandon Rypeon, Joanne Spielman, Meg Edson, Mark Stoefels, Pete Vlantis, Stacey Forman, Susie Tapiero, Jim Wyzard, Karin Stover, Nancy McCarthy, Nancy Hamilton, Kim Gooz, Max Helfgott, and Cathy Fowler. Kevin Maselka of Planet Fitness was a great host in the formative stage of this book. Samantha Karinch shared home and car to help us bridge the distance between us. FILA Corporation created and contributed great clothing that stands up to abuse from us fitness nuts who wear it with pride. Last but absolutely not least, we want to thank our moms, dads, brothers and sisters for lovingly kicking us in the butt all these years, and thank you, God, for the opportunities to design our dreams and live them to the fullest.

Sarge and Krunchie

For all those who try, tried, and thought they'd died—keep on! And for our families, who love us no matter how wacky we are.

INTRODUCTION

Dear Reader,

You are ready for this book if your body offends you. You have found your humiliation threshold. Maybe you reached it when your beeper went off and someone yelled, "He's backing up!" Maybe you reached it when someone mooed as your big ol' butt waddled down the street. Or worst of all, when you tried to run across a parking lot someone yelled, "STAMPEDE!"

So you've come to me to make a change. You told me your gut's growing and your can is the size of Kansas. Now, I'll bet you're going to tell me you don't like exercise and want me to make you like it. Well, fragile reader, before we can know whether or not that's possible, I have to ask you two questions: What makes you think I can help you? And, if I were to tell you I can't do anything for you, how would you feel? Don't blow this second question off and go on to the next sentence. Answer it. If we are going to make any progress here, you have to trust my lead. Well, how would you feel if I told you I can't help. Discouraged? My goal in saying that is not to make you feel discouraged. It's to let you know that none of this is up to me. It's up to you, but you'd better *believe* I'll help just as I've helped thousands of other people over the past fifteen years get in the best condition of their lives.

It started in the early 1980s, when I was a dental technician in the Navy, but my love was fitness. Wherever I was stationed, I begged to be involved in the command (base or ship) fitness programs, which were, for the most part, underfunded and ignored. In boot camp, I was the athletic petty officer, which means I was tasked to assemble a group of smelly, homesick recruits and lead them through a basic fitness program. Then, after the crash course that made me a dental technician, it was off to the aircraft carrier *USS Carl Vinson,* where I served on the ship's gym advisory council. Sounds important, huh? Funny thing was that the people on the ship who really cared about the gym were the Marines; almost none of the sailors hefted weights. So, I became a mate of the squared-away, buzz-cut Marines. We had to really *want* to work out, too. First of all, it took a lot of patience to wait between the ship's rolls to do a bench press. Some exercises were out of the question while we were underway—if you did them, you might eat iron. Most important, the hot, stinky gym, which was located at the rear end of the ship called the fantail, did nothing to inspire people.

Imagine you're with me. We're on an aircraft carrier one deck below the landing area for the jets. Here we are, cramped in this tiny room, with egos that need the fuel of an F14, and aircraft landing fifteen feet overhead every ninety seconds. Our junky equipment must have been donated by some middle school in East Hallelujah. There is no air-conditioning or even air circulation. But do we complain? Heck, no. We're eighteen years old, cooped up and more grateful than you can imagine to be saved from *Gilligan's Island* reruns.

I *wanted* to be there—that's what made it great.

That dedication has only gotten more powerful for me. And now, at Boot Camp, I have found my passion: To drive huff-and-puffin' recruits like you to rediscover how to have fun with your bodies. After that, fitness, energy, and greater mental alertness happen before you know it.

I look at it quite simply. If you can *enjoy* exercising and eating right, you *will* exercise and eat right. That's what I am going to help you do—enjoy the process of getting healthier. Hopefully, I will (literally) have you laughing your butt off. Think about it. If you were (or are) a smoker, it's hard as heck to quit. I read a report that said it's easier to quit heroin than smoking. That's tough, but you can do it without patches or pills or any other crutch if you enjoy the process.

Boot Camp is not about deprivation—it's about fun. I am going to assign you crazy, hilarious, wacky ways to get yourself healthy and fit, and we are going to have a blast. I am going to give you opportunities to E-mail me personally with your challenges and work with others throughout the book. This is going to be like no other book you have ever read or any other program you have tried. Strap on your seat belt and fire up your high beams: The Sarge is going to get your behind in shape.

Now, let's go!

The Sarge

CHAPTER ONE
WHAT'S IN IT FOR YOU?

Listen up. We're looking for a few fat men and women! We want you!

You and only you are responsible for your health, but you might need someone to help you hold yourself accountable. No, this is not the government's new healthcare program. Uncle Sam is not going to give you a tax credit for exercising. You *are* going to get daily help from the Sarge if—and only if—you do your part.

You can laugh, close the book, or just plain ignore me if you choose, but the bottom line is that you picked up this book for a reason; and the reason is probably that you have let your body turn into a gelatinous blob, or you're not even able to walk up a flight of stairs without risk of a coronary. Have I struck a nerve? Did I hit home? Are your feelings hurt? One thing is for sure: I have your attention. A second thing is for sure: You found the right guy to help you out.

The first difference between the Boot Camp program and a health club or the dumbbells in your closet is that I will help hold you accountable to yourself—and to me.

The second difference is that I will help make exercise fun. You get to play with the real GI Joe and you WILL enjoy it.

The third difference is that you can and will do every exercise in Boot Camp, no matter how unfit you are, unless you have a serious physical condition that requires medical supervision or you are totally lazy.

As you flip through this book you will see pictures of folks of all shapes and sizes. All of them are our daily victims. That's right, *no models*. Two of the biggest guys, Frank and Charles, are best buddies. The day we did the test photographs (to see who would be in the book) we naturally picked them. We scheduled the photo shoots three weeks after the test shots were done. In those three weeks, Frank and Charles went through Boot Camp with one of my instructors. I didn't see them that whole time, so when they showed up for the shoot, I couldn't believe my eyes. These two bloated, jolly jelly doughnuts had dropped eighten to twenty pounds each! *Each!* So don't even think you can't do this program or that you won't see amazing results—you can and you will.

You can expect to lose 5 to 7 percent of your blubber body during your three weeks in Boot Camp. So if you're a 150-pound woman, you could drop eight to ten pounds. Men, if your 200-pound bodies do a few push-ups and you keep the beer to a minimum, you could see ten to fourteen pounds come off. The Boot Camp record is twenty-four pounds, but it was set by a very big boy. Don't try to beat his number, just pay attention to your own body.

Would you get results like that from wandering into a gym? Ha! Picture this: You go to a health club. You walk in there and fiddle-fart around with a couple machines, and then the confusion sets in. "Why are the guys prettier than the girls, and how do those guys get such a close shave on their legs?" you ask yourself. And those aerobics classes—heck, man, do you dance like I do? It's bad enough I can't dance, but to wear an outfit that has every ass dimple showing while I gyrate and hop is too much for me. And what about those machines? You need a degree in computer science or mechanical engineering to figure them out. AAAAGGGHHH!! So you scratch your rear end and leave. If you don't go back, who cares? On the other hand, if you use Boot Camp to jump-start your attitude as well as your butt, you'll have a blast and will learn to care. I am going to kick you in the ass and hold your hand at the same time.

By the time you master the exercises in this book—and that includes the exercise of eating decent food—your mind will have mastered a few things, too. It will drive your body toward better health as effectively as it used to hold you back. Other incredible things will happen at the same time: You'll feel proud at the sight of your shrinking gut and butt in the mirror. You'll feel sexier. You'll think The Sarge is one helluva guy. I am a helluva guy!

How did I get to be this way? For starters, as I told you in the In-

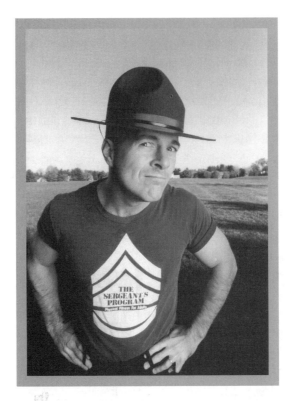

troduction, Uncle Sam sent me out to sea. It was like some voice from above boomed: "Mr. Avon, can you hang on to your sense of humor when you're dreaming of girls, but wake up to a ship full of farting, spitting sailors and crop-topped Marines?" I yelled back, "Yes, Sir," then proceeded to knock myself out in the ship's gym. After my buddy Terry and I set up the weights so they wouldn't fall off the barbell when the ship listed, we started training people. What began as diversion became a profession. Now it's a passion, as well as a career, and *you* get to share it, recruit.

Starting out Boot Camp, you will be excited. I want you to keep that energy high every day of the program, and there are two big ways to do it.

First, do the mental exercises in this book, not just the physical ones. Some of them are wacko to the tenth degree, but they will help you break nasty habits, especially the eating ones. We have to get a little crazy to help you eyeball your bad habits and understand how much they hold you back. And, as I said before, you will have fun on this journey, but you will also get results! You have my word. Would I lie to you?

Second, make this a team effort—you, me, and whomever else you can drag along. Personally, I recommend that the whole family go through Boot Camp together—at least the eating part—or buy this book for a buddy or two. Then you can all kick each other in the rear as you go through Boot Camp together. Another way to fight the urge for a fistful of French fries is to visit www.sarge.com. And you'll hear from me on that site, so watch out.

You will begin Boot Camp with an aggressive commitment to changing your body. It comes from having an image of what you want to look and feel like, what you want to see in the mirror, and how you'll feel when you roll out of bed in the morning. Understand two things:

1. *You will feel better immediately.* About a year ago, I had a meeting with corporate executives about doing a fitness and wellness program for their senior staff. I have never seen a more stressful environment in my life. I have been in divorced households signing someone up for the program; I have been in corporations going bankrupt and in Fortune 500 corporations that had layoffs when their quarterly returns slumped. Never have I seen this level of stress. On Day One of their Boot Camp program, they all laughed at themselves and each other. They smiled, felt good, cracked jokes, and couldn't wait until the next session. Their company paid for three sessions a week, but many of them signed up for optional nutrition programs. They felt good! Sure, they couldn't walk down the street in a midriff-cut shirt without getting a chuckle, but they felt healthy, which is more important than just looking perfect. Yes, they did lose fat, but that was secondary to their immediate gains in energy, self-esteem, and fun.

2. *Your expectations may be high and you may never achieve them; but stay on course and you will come very close.* Have you ever heard the saying, "Shoot for the stars and you might get to the moon?" That's probably what's going to happen, because fitness is not a destination, it is a journey.

You will have rewards along the way, though. You'll feel the satis-faction of your efforts—less jiggle when you walk, more energy when you play with your spouse. In Boot Camp, you will learn to set achievable fitness goals, then surprise yourself by exceeding them. Your goal for the first three weeks may be to just jog around the block, for example, but after six months, you may be ready for a 5K (3.1-mile) race. Your first goal for that race may be to finish it, but two months later, your goal may be to complete it in thirty min-utes. Eventually, you might be able to run a marathon like other graduates of Boot Camp. Ninety percent of these people who are running 26.2 miles couldn't see their toes, let alone touch them, when they first came to Boot Camp. Running a marathon might not be your objective, though. You might just want to fit into pants you wore last year. Once you accomplish that, who knows? Maybe you'll decide to be a competitive athlete. Remember: Shoot for the stars. David Brooks, the man who did all the photographs for this book, started out in Boot Camp as a pudgy guy. Here he is five years later racing bicycles and with less than 10 percent body fat! Your goals will change all the time, so keep an open mind. Each time you progress from goal to goal, you will be moving forward—that's fitness.

I have seen thousands of people slam their butts on a stair-climber machine and burn five hundred calories a day for the sole satisfaction of squeezing into a smaller pair of jeans. Ask Oprah Winfrey what happened when she tried that approach. She reports that within days of the big squeeze, she couldn't fit into those jeans anymore, then her weight shot up to more than two hundred pounds again. During this yo-yoing, she went to a boxing match be-tween Mike Tyson and Tyrell Biggs and realized her weight was the same as Tyson's.[1] The talk show queen of the world weighed the same as the Heavyweight Champion of the World! It was an unfor-gettable moment that stung her and helped her set fitness goals and stick with them. Way to go, Oprah! Take a lesson: If your only goal is to fit into a smaller dress or jeans, it's a shortsighted goal that will not help you get fit.

[1] Bob Greene and Oprah Winfrey, *Make the Connection* (Hyperion, 1996), 10.

Boot Camp is not about looking sexy in a bathing suit or a tight pair of pants. It's about having fun with fitness—like a kid—and being healthy.

Remember when you were little and liked to go out and play all the time and run to your friend's house? You never used a car. You used your legs and a bicycle to get places and thought that was *fun*. My goal is to help you have that kind of fun again. I want to help you bring back your joy of movement.

The journey starts here. *Boot Camp* is a three-week program that starts out slowly so you don't burn out. I kick you in the seat of your pants at the same time I hold your hand and make you laugh. Am I a drill instructor? Not really. Am I tough? Tough enough. Have I killed anybody? Not yet. Am I going to start with you? I doubt it. Are you going to have fun? You bet your excess baggage!

Boot Camp is basic exercise that you can do anywhere: This is a no-frills, no-expense, no-gym, no-spandex, three-week program. You can report for duty at home, on vacation, and maybe even on your lunch hour at work. You will take this program with you wherever you go. For the next twenty-one days, this is the bible for your body.

What are you going to do? Brisk walking that may turn into jogging, believe it or not. You will do push-ups. Some of you will start on your knees, then progress to your toes. You will do dips to get rid of "Bingo" arms. (Haven't you seen those old ladies raising their arms to yell "BINGO!" and that big flap of skin is flopping like a turkey neck?) You will do abdominal crunches designed to strengthen the part that hangs over your belt. You will do the superman to strengthen your lower back and rear end. You will do other exercises to burn lots of calories and fat. And you will stretch, stretch, stretch.

Will you be a little sore after exercise? What do you think? Will you find it a little difficult to do the exercises the next day? Yyyyyes. Do you want to get in shape? Of course! In order to condition a muscle you have to stress it each and every time. And to stress it means you put a little more load on it than you think it can handle. That means if you did three push-ups a day this week, you will do four a day next week.

At this point, you might be saying to yourself, "I wish I could get rid of my bingo arms," or "I wish I could do ten sit-ups without feeling like I was going to bust a hemorrhoid." Great! Welcome to Boot Camp: *Be all you want to be.*

Or, are you saying to yourself, "I used to be able to do twenty-five push-ups in thirty seconds. I used to bench-press my body weight." Great! Welcome to Boot Camp: *Be all you used to be.*

We want a few *good* men and women. We want YOU!

CHAPTER TWO
REPORT FOR DUTY, FAT ASS

Strip down, recruit! You are about to take your fitness physical for Boot Camp. That's right, tests. The only way to assess your fitness level is to test your big behind. Are you ready for these tests? Are you ready for me? After you yell, "YES, SIR!" ask your doctor. I haven't lost anyone yet, and I'm not about to start with you.

By "doctor" I don't mean someone you trust like your chiropractor, acupuncturist, or mother. No, I don't have any problem with them. I visit a chiropractor regularly and think the others have a place in life, too. Right now, though, you need to see an MD who administers traditional tests to find out if your heart and lungs have holes in them. If your legs look like something in a Colonel Sanders bucket and you've been turning your butt into cottage cheese for the past few years, you need to have a complete physical examination to find out if there is any reason why you cannot or should not do the exercises in this book. That, my little French fry, is an order.

Here's what makes up the Boot Camp entrance exam: *body-fat measurement, aerobic endurance, muscle endurance, flexibility*, and one funky haircut. Your gear list is as follows:

1. A seamstress tape measure (Use cloth, not metal, unless you want scars.)
2. A scale (Don't buy one, borrow it for the test, because you won't need it during Boot Camp.)
3. No. 2 pencils (It's a test, got it?)
4. A one-mile flat walking path (You can measure this in your car or waste fifteen dollars on a pacing device.)

Do your tests in the following order—that's my order, not your order. There's a reason: Do it my way and you stay warmed up so you don't hurt yourself. If you have to take a break between tests, pay attention: "Warmed up" means you have perspiration on your forehead, or at the very least, you have done *something* for five minutes that raised your heart rate. (You don't have to tell me what it was.)

BODY-FAT MEASUREMENT

Did you hear me? I said, "Strip down!" Now grab your tape measure and hit the scale.

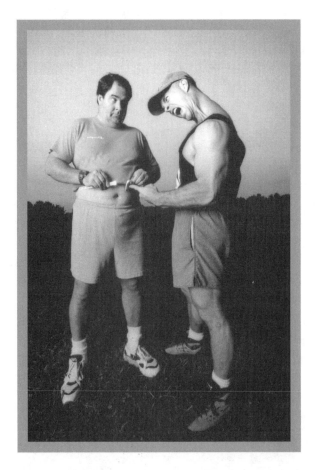

Show me the fat! Accurate starting measurements help you build fitness goals.

Men

1. Record your height in inches.
2. Put your naked behind on the scale and record the result.
3. Have someone help you measure the following body parts. Take each measurement twice and record the average.
   - Neck: Put the tape around your neck at the Adam's apple. Don't pull it so tight that you gag or your skin is indented.
   - Abdominal area: Clean the lint out of your belly button. Encircle your waist at navel level. Make sure the tape covers those love handles. The tape should not make a dent in the skin, but it should fit the skin tightly.

Subtract your neck measurement from your abdominal measurement. Unless you're the star of a circus side show, the number will be in the double digits. Go directly to the body-fat grid in the back of this book (Appendix A); don't stop to look at the pictures. Across the top of the grid, find your height. On the left side, find the number you got by subtracting neck from waist inches. The number in that column is an approximation of your percentage of body fat. For you young soldiers with monosyllabic vocabularies, that means it isn't exact. The number could be off by 3 percent, one way or the other. More important than accuracy is the fact that this is your "starting number"; in three weeks, you will contrast your new results with it.

Women

1. Record your height in inches.
2. Put your naked body on a scale and record the result.
3. See the instructions above on technique. Measure your neck, abdominal area, and hips at the widest point. To make sure you get this right, put your feet together and point them forward while your best friend, who would never tell a soul about this, measures your buttocks and vicinity. You want to be sure to capture the widest part of your hips, so several measurements may be necessary. Measure each of the three areas twice and record the average.

Women, you have a little more mental work than the men to calculate body fat. Begin by adding your waist and hip measurements.

Sounds bad so far, doesn't it? Now subtract the circumference of your neck. You'll get a much larger number than the guys; but your grid is different, so it doesn't matter.

Give me real weight, not driver's-license weight. It is not our main focus anyway; we're looking at losing inches.

Do not obsess about the numbers on the scale. When someone meets you, do you think that person mutters, "Gee, I'll bet she

One woman who turned in her paperwork for Boot Camp listed her weight as 145. I took one look at her and thought, "Uh, uh." I put her on a scale and got a result that didn't surprise me, but it apparently surprised her: 198 pounds. She said to me, "Oh, dear! My scale must be off!" Either that, or she ate one jumbo pizza last night.

weighs a good 148." No, it's "Hey now!" or "Good Lord!" All a scale does is measure weight, not what you are made of; it does not give an accurate reading of your health or fitness. Your tape measure will continue to be a more useful tool.

When you drop fifteen pounds of fat and gain five pounds of muscle, the scale will show a ten-pound decrease, *and* your girth will be reduced. For a 200-pound person, that could represent a loss of several inches at the waist. What does that mean, math wiz? It means *muscle weighs more than fat* and the scale is very misleading. Losing fifteen pounds of fat is great, and gaining five pounds of muscle is even better. The muscle gain gives you a stronger body and more active metabolism, that is, one that burns calories more efficiently. So, after your initial weigh-in, trash the scale and stick with a tape measure.

AEROBIC ENDURANCE

Determine your resting heart rate. Here's how: Two days in a row, just as you wake up, lightly touch your carotid pulse (see photo) and take your heart rate for sixty seconds. Don't fall back to sleep while you're doing this! And don't do this after a dirty dream! The result should be roughly the same for the two days, and the average is your resting heart rate. If there is a wide spread, say, ten beats or more per minute, either you didn't do it correctly or didn't listen to my orders regarding the dream.

Now that you know your resting heart rate, where do you fit on

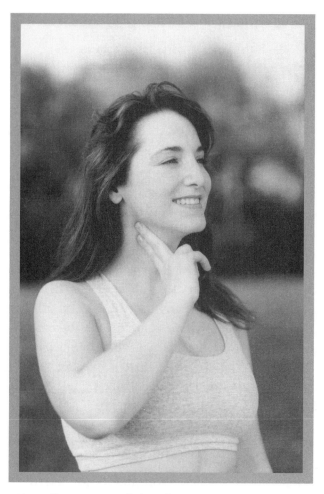

Keep the pressure light when you take your pulse.

the scale below? If you are off the chart (off the bottom of the chart, that is), make sure your doctor knows it.

Take your blood pressure. You can do this at your local drugstore

BEATS PER MINUTE	
Excellent	<55
Good	55-64
Average	65-72
Fair	73-80
Poor	>80

Note: The same numbers apply to both genders

or doctor's office, or you can buy your own blood pressure cuff for about twenty-five dollars. Follow the directions. If you're carrying a lot of extra fat, go to your doctor and don't bother to buy the cuff. A standard-size blood-pressure cuff will give you an elevated reading and that won't help you at all. Record the numbers. They'll make more sense later.

Drive your car one-half mile in a flat area free of flying debris such as bullets and bird turds. Tie a yellow ribbon on a tree to remind yourself where the half-mile point is.

Turn your car around, drive it back to the starting point, and park it. Get out and walk your one-mile course as briskly as possible without killing yourself. At any time, if your breathing gets out of control, slow down. Ideally, you should walk the entire mile, but if you can go only half a mile, then do that (and take a cab back and try again tomorrow). The second your foot hits the last step of the course, take your heart rate for sixty seconds. This is your exercise heart rate.

Subtract your age from 220; the result is your maximum heart rate. How close were you to that number after your walking test? If you were close—let's say 80 percent or more—then keep walking in Boot Camp and save the jogging for later. So, if you're forty years old, and your heart rate after the test was 150, don't run unless you have a Rottweiler on your tail. Wait until your heart rate is around

125 after a mile walk before you blast off. There's another way of measuring your cardio fitness that I like better, but it involves math. If you have a calculator and can handle the big numbers, turn to Appendix B.

You can also do this test by cycling or swimming a set distance. Of course, if you could swim half a mile, you probably wouldn't be reading this book. Whatever you do, be sure your activity lasts about the same length of time as a one-mile walk—about fifteen to twenty minutes. The important thing is that you use the same activity and measuring device now and at the end of Boot Camp, so we can quantify your improvement.

SUMMARY: AEROBIC ENDURANCE TEST

1. Take your resting heart rate. Record it and check the grid.
2. Take your blood pressure. Record it.
3. Walk a mile as briskly as you can. Slow down if you have difficulty breathing. Record how long it took and what your heart rate was after you stopped. To get a measure of your oxygen consumption, turn to the grid in Appendix B.

MUSCLE ENDURANCE

Endurance is the ability to move an object repeatedly, like carrying two grocery bags up three flights of stairs with your keys clenched in your teeth and trying to open the door before the dog runs out. In this section of your Boot Camp entrance exam, you will test the endurance of muscles, starting with your upper body—chest, arms, and shoulders.

I saw an eighty-plus-year-old woman walking down the street with two grocery bags. My instinct was to be a gentleman and carry the bags. Wrong! She was not struggling; she needs to do this to stay strong. Help like that makes people helpless. So next time you see a Boy Scout, straighten him out. And the next time you see an old lady, have her carry your stuff and tell her Sarge says it's for her own good. She'll thank me someday (I think).

Upper Body

A push-up does not look like you're humping the ground. In a proper push-up, your nose, nipples, and navel touch the ground at the same time. If you happen to be more gifted in the navel, lose weight. If your nipples scrape the dirt first, buy a good sports bra. If your nose hits before the other body parts, it's going to hurt.

The details on push-up form are covered in chapter 6. Although this is not a test of form, but one of endurance, always try to align your body properly to prevent injury. Keep the nose-nipples-navel guidance in mind. If you do the push-ups on your knees rather than your toes—a modified push-up—cross your ankles, bring your heels into the butt, and make sure your can isn't in the air.

A new recruit came to our offices to take her Boot Camp test. I said, "Give me as many push-ups as you can." She pumped them out, one after the other, then suddenly stopped. I said, "What are you doing? I can tell you have more in you!" "It hurts," she replied. In fact, she didn't hurt at all; she was just tired and bored. Because she didn't do regular exercise, though, she did not know how to differentiate between pain and fatigue. When she started to sweat, she thought she had a problem. In other words, she had just started to feel the exercise when she quit.

There's a lesson in this, recruit: Health and fitness are about progression, not maintenance. If you only do as many repetitions as you can until you start to feel the exercise, you will not progress. You must push *beyond* that point. Get used to it now!

A few recruits may find that a push-up on the toes or the knees is too tough to do. Unless you have a damaged rotator cuff (a group of small shoulder muscles) or other injury, the weakness could be in your head. Don't give me any lame-butt excuse either! I had a sixty-year-old woman from the garden club of a posh suburb approach me about training. (This tree-lined neighborhood is where the trainers work out for the clients.) She told me she couldn't do push-ups while she was doing them. So spare me your whining and hit the deck, soldier. You'd better try before you proceed to the last resort.

By the way, I am not picking on any particular socioeconomic group. Mentioning the woman's neighborhood lets me make the point that when people abandon manual labor—whether or not they can afford to—they have to find other ways to incorporate vigorous movement into their lives. People all over the country spend good money on ways to avoid cleaning, gardening, and shoveling snow, then get sick of how they look and pay people like me more good money to make them move.

Back to push-ups. (You thought I forgot, didn't you?) If you

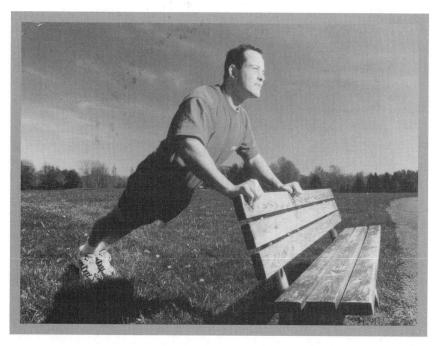

If you absolutely can't do this, then do your pushup against the wall.

have really tried and still found yourself eating carpet fibers on the first regular push-up, do your push-ups against the wall, or by pushing off a countertop or sturdy bench (see photo). Put your feet about three to four feet away from the wall and your hands directly in front of your shoulders. Point your fingertips upward. Put your nose and chest to the wall at the same time; keep your legs locked.

For the test, do as many push-ups as you can in two minutes. If at any time you have to stop, mark down how many you did. In other words, you have no rest breaks, pauses, or lapses of consciousness in this test. As soon as you stop or break your rhythm, you're done. You can go as fast or slow as you like, but you must be consistent.

SUMMARY: MUSCLE ENDURANCE TEST FOR THE UPPER BODY

Do as many push-ups as you can in two minutes.

Begin with a standard push-up, if you can do it, then drop to a modified push-up if you must. If you have a hard time with either, do push-ups against a wall, or using a countertop or bench.

FLEXIBILITY

You need to be warmed up for this test, so if you were a slacker after the push-ups, move around and get a little perspiration on your forehead before you take it.

Sit on the ground with your legs in front of you and about twelve inches apart. Tape a yardstick to the ground in front of you, with "0" toward your body and your heels at the fifteen-inch mark. Take a seamstress (cloth) tape measure and lay it perpendicular to the yardstick at your feet. (See photo.) Put one hand over the other so your middle fingers overlap, then, as you lean forward to do a toe-touch, slide the tape measure as far as possible with your fingertips. Notice I said "slide," not "bounce and shove." Be sure to drop your head between your arms so you have a comfortable stretch from your tail bone to

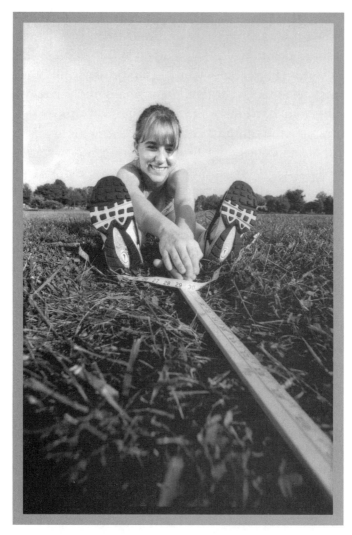

Be sure you're warmed up to take this test.
And no bouncing—I'm watching!

your head bone. Mark down the number on the yardstick that the tape measure reached. Do it again, then average the two and record the result.

At the end of this chapter, there is one measure of how well you did—100 percent meaning "that's as good as it gets unless you're an Olympic gymnast." If you want to see how well you fare in your own age group, turn to Appendix C.

Abdominal Area

If you have a bad back, or you're prone to muscle spasms in the back, or your doctor suggests you don't do this, don't do this.

Put the soles of your feet together in a butterfly sitting position. Have someone anchor your feet, or put them under a couch if they fit. Keeping your back straight, do as many sit-ups as you can in two minutes. Come up to the point where your elbows touch your knees. Do not interlock your fingers behind your head; your arms must be folded across your chest. The first time your elbows do not touch your knees, stop. You're done.

Get the body position for this test right, recruit! In the old days, when Sarge was a lowly private, we did sit-ups with straight legs, and that's probably how you learned to do them, too. Then a couple years ago, some brilliant exercise physiologist like Mark Occhipinti at American Fitness Professionals and Associates realized that we were only using hip flexors by doing it that way; our abs were just going along for the ride. If you raise your legs high like you're marching in the Rose Bowl Parade, you do the same thing. In order to disengage those strong hip muscles and work the abs you must sit in the butterfly position. Mark recently introduced the Marines to this technique, so consider yourself up to date with the fighting elite.

SUMMARY: THE *BOOT CAMP* PHYSICAL TESTS

- Take weight, height, and body measurements.
- Do a brisk one-mile walk.
- Do some kind of push-up for two minutes straight.
- Record how far you pushed a tape measure up the yardstick between your legs.
- Do as many sit-ups as you can in two minutes.

With your test results in front of you, look at this chart,[1] but don't obsess on the rankings. You're in Boot Camp because you

[1] Courtesy of ARA/Human Factors.

need to make a change, so you are not going to be in the performance range of elite athletes. In fact, you may be somewhere near
"0." So what? Just *don't stay there!*

At the end of three weeks, you will do tests like this again to see
how much Boot Camp has improved your body-fat measurement,
aerobic endurance, muscle endurance, and flexibility. Your mind
will be blown with your progress! You will look as good as you did in
real boot camp the first time (or Canada).

PERCENTILE RANKINGS FOR SELECTED FITNESS TESTS

%	RHR[2] (BPM)	% Fat	Push-ups	Sit-ups	Sit & reach
100	39	<8	82	100	24
90	56	10.3	41	64	19.1
80	61	12.7	36	57	17.1
70	64	14.6	32	52	17.1
60	68	16.2	30	49	16.3
50	71	17.7	27	44	15.3
40	74	19.0	25	42	14.6
30	79	20.8	21	36	13.7
20	83	23.4	19	30	12
10	92	26.8	14	25	10.2
0	100	42.2	0	0	0

[2]Resting Heart Rate (beats per minute)

CHAPTER THREE
THE CHOW HALL: DON'T EAT WITHOUT THINKING

For this chapter, you will need a log book at all times. Fill in the answers to *all* the questions—no answers, no diploma. And remember: If you lie, I will have to kill you.

Take a camera and your log book and go to your refrigerator. If you are 100 percent committed to changing, take your videocam and shoot your entire refrigerator, pantry, and shelves. You can actually record the growth of mold on your bologna. It's a horror movie and it's all yours! Remember: "You are what you eat."

Open your refrigerator and take a picture of every splattered shelf, every sticky bin, every box of frozen pizza. No "Ha, ha, Sarge"—do it! Put the pictures in your log book for future guilt. Log everything you see. If you don't know what something is, save the picture, but throw the real thing away.

Now you're ready to learn.

What time is it? If you're starting your day right by waking up to The Sarge, then grab a big bowl of cereal or oatmeal and dump some low-fat milk and fresh fruit on it. Now listen up and chow down, 'cuz this is going to be the toughest chapter of the book for you.

Why? Because at some point, someone told you it was okay to eat garbage. (Maybe that person was you, young soldier.) You gave yourself permission to shovel chicken wings and onion rings down your throat. By the way, have you ever watched someone eat a plate of nachos like it was their last supper? That slimy cheese product drips down their chins, and the sour cream goes up their nose.

Yummy, huh? They're totally out of control and careless. That's YOU, and your bad habits have caught up with you. You're as big as a house and slow as a turtle, but there's hope: You have given *me* the task of undoing your lousy conditioning. Of course, you expect me to fix you in one measly chapter. Surprise—I will! But you better believe your slackin' can is not going to sit back and enjoy my barking orders. You are going to get off your La-Z-Boy, turn off your eight-track tape deck, forget Richard Simmons (I am his evil twin), and go to work. Now, let's kick the tires and light the fires: From here on in, I'm in charge.

WATER

Your body is nearly 70 percent water. The earth is nearly 70 percent water. When the earth doesn't get enough water, living things die. Get the message? Keep your cells alive! I drink a gallon a day; that's sixteen eight-ounce glasses if you use a glass (I don't). I dare you to match me.

If you are not up to it, fine. I'm not going to tell you to bloat yourself. Our strategy is different. Along with your water, you're going to drink real juice and eat a lot of water-rich foods. You'll know you are on the right track if your urine is always clear. That's right, I want to see clear urine every day, every time. And I will check.

Clear pee pee! Clear pee pee! Clear pee pee!

Here are the rules:

- The water should be pure. Depending on where you live, that may rule out anything your pipes touch.
- The juice should be fresh. And I mean fresh, not the grocery store sugar-loaded kids' stuff. Check the labels on bottled and canned juices to see why. A lot of "juices" contain sweeteners and traces of things that come from chemistry labs, not from fruits or vegetables.

LISTEN UP!

To help get water-rich foods in your diet, always eat a salad with dinner.

• Since your body is nearly 70 percent water—you guessed it—70 percent of what you eat should be water-rich. Potato chips are not a water-rich food. Oranges and lettuce and grapes and green beans are water-rich foods; they cleanse your body and send vitamins to your cells. A lime is water-rich, but its value is lost when it's in a margarita.

You may be feeling insubordinate right now. You may be thinking, "French fries are made out of potato and that's a vegetable, so they're water-rich." Fine, Ricky Recruit. Just hang on to that delusion while you do these assignments—I dare you! Your big ol' butt will stay that way, this book will end up a coaster on your table, and when your friends come over they will laugh at you 'cuz you ate your way through Boot Camp. So cut the crap and get crackin'.

ASSIGNMENT ONE

Go to a fast-food restaurant (aka fat-food restaurant). You are about to do investigative research. No, I'm not kidding. You're about to have a lot of fun at other people's expense, especially if you do this with a buddy.

Park your car in the lot, or sit outside on a bench. Observe twenty people and jot down in your log book what you notice about them. Record the answers to these questions:

1. How many are overweight?
2. How many are grossly overweight (i.e., fatter than you are)?
3. Where is the focus of each person headed toward the door of the restaurant:
   A. on the door (meaning, they can't wait to get in)
   B. on their cash (meaning, they have to know how much they can afford)
   C. on their kids, or each other (meaning, this is an outing, not a routine)
4. If you were going into the restaurant right now, what would you order?
5. When these twenty people come out, how many are carrying
   A. a large greasy bag, with a large drink?
   B. a medium greasy bag, with a medium drink?
   C. a small greasy bag (or no bag), with a drink?

6. How often does the size of the bag match the amount of fat on the body?

7. How many of them chomped on their food before they got back to the car? (You got the picture: Waddling slob with fistful of French fries tries to open car door; keys slip out of greasy hands, cussing follows.)

8. Now go into the restaurant. Listen to what twenty people order.

9. How many of them bought a salad? (meaning, either their kids dragged them here and they are desperately trying to find something edible, or they are trying to make a change)

10. How many added a large order of fries to the meal? (meaning, they don't give a damn)

11. How many got a double-blob meal, like a double cheeseburger? (meaning, see above)

12. How many of them ordered a diet drink with their "fat meals"? (meaning, a part of them wants to make a change—there's hope!)

13. Take a whiff of the oil in the French fryer. Inhale that aroma of fatty meat burning on a greasy grill. As your lungs and throat fill with the stinking, scorching grease and your hair absorbs the nasty stench, look at the zitty-faced kids who make that food and look at the bellies of the people who shove it in their mouths without even breathing. REREAD THIS PARAGRAPH FIVE TIMES BEFORE YOU GO TO THE NEXT QUESTION and think about this: If you were to videotape these people eating and play it back for them, would they be embarrassed? Would they be offended?

14. Now what do you want to order? (It's okay to say "Nothing, Sarge.")

15. Is it any different from what you would have ordered before you thought about it?

This may sound wacky, but if you commit to the above assignment you will be shocked at the results and laugh your tail off. You will be happy to know that I have converted thousands of victims to the sport of watching other people eat. Miss Manners would call this rude; I call it Step One.

Before I go to the next assignment, let me confess. I used to be one of the people you're looking at. No, I never had a weight problem, but I ate that junk and felt like doo-doo for hours. I did it for years, then one day I stopped the habit. I found myself tired right after lunch. I needed a nap! I gave it some hard thought (about one second), and from that day forward I quit eating garbage. Do I slip up and order too much cheese on my pizza? Do I stop thinking long enough to eat too many Christmas cookies? Do I ever eat too fast? Sure I do, but it doesn't happen on a regular basis. That's the difference—it's not habit anymore.

ASSIGNMENT TWO

Go to a nice restaurant. Does that mean fast-food joints aren't "nice"? What do you think, buttnut?

Once again, observe twenty people and jot down in your log book what you notice about them. Record the answers to these nine questions:

1. How many people come dressed to expand? (muumuus, spandex, no belt . . .)
2. How many people treat their vegetables like an ugly date?
3. How many people spoon fat on their potato?
4. How many people order stuff with cream sauce?
5. How many people eat a gloppy dessert?
6. How many people have their salad dressing put on the side?
7. How many people trim the fat off their meat?
8. How many people take the skin off their chicken?
9. How many people limit themselves to what they want and either take the rest in a doggy bag or leave it on the plate?

LISTEN UP!

To avoid eating junk or overeating at a restaurant, have a tall glass of H_2O and eat a little of your own food before you go. And always keep a large (full) water bottle in your car. You'll reduce the temptation to pig out while you save money.

The first five address the habits of fat-assed frogs; they probably even look like the Budweiser mascots. The last four give you hints. Yes, you can enter a restaurant hungry and leave full of energy, instead of rolling out the door like a bloated disaster looking for a bathroom.

This next exercise was a shocker for me and it probably will be for you.

ASSIGNMENT THREE

1. Go to your favorite restaurant. It doesn't matter if it's a "nice" one or not. Go to the back entrance. You know, it's the place with the puddles of used dishwater.
2. What do you see?
3. What do you smell?
4. Would you describe the environment as "sanitary"?

Let me make you sick. When I did this assignment, I went to my favorite local restaurant, one that I thought was clean. I discovered that their method of drying fish was hanging it over a dumpster out back. No, I am not kidding; they hung fish to dry over the garbage. Did I hear you say, "yeeechk!"? My reaction precisely. Now you know why they no longer have me as a customer.

You want to make sure that whatever goes in your body comes from a clean place and stays clean while it's being prepared. It's all part of the regimen of keeping your body clean, that is, in a state where it's using fat for energy, not accumulating it.

Over the years, you've probably become saturated with information about good eating. Why haven't you used it? You have to want to use it. If you really want to do something, you will, recruit! And if you did your assignments, I'll bet my stripes you're closer to "wanting to" than you were before.

Now, let me give you another powerful reason to want to change your diet: self-control.

A steady diet of food and drink with a high sugar content will affect your ability to manage your emotions. It will upset your good sense to the point where you might say "Scrap this good-diet crap.

Dump the Sarge." And if I ever hear you think that, recruit, you'd better hide in that slimy refrigerator of yours!

At least for the time you are in Boot Camp—a measly three weeks—you *must* reduce your intake of sugar. If you do go over the edge, go to the Boot Camp site at www.sarge.com for a dose of inspiration. I will not let you eat garbage! Garbage is for maggots!

BODY POLLUTION

Speaking of garbage, it's time to tell you ugly stories about calcium propionate and fat birds.

I will point my finger straight at your drooling mouth and tell you that, with only a few exceptions, food additives, including preservatives, have no place in a live human body. Your digestive tract, liver, kidney, and other organs have to work overtime to remove that junk from your system. Monosodium glutamate and Red Dye no. 3 are fine for lab experiments on rats, but I accept no rats in my Boot Camp.

Here's the possible exception: Some so-called food additives are actually vitamins put in your milk and cereal to boost the nutritional value. For example, d-alpha tocopherol is one of the substances that makes up vitamin E. Don't make the mistake of thinking that extra vitamins will help you get through Boot Camp, though. Your body works to eliminate whatever it doesn't need; save that energy for push-ups.

You'll find preservatives in anything that's designed to hang around for a long time. If you're over forty, you may remember the stacks of well-preserved food that mom stored in the basement in case a nuclear attack prevented the family from going outside for a decade. Somebody should have told mom that a steady diet of that crap would kill you if the radiation didn't. And what about those canned goodies? There are vitamins in those vegetables, but they diminish over time. Those cans have a shelf life, so you should dump your emergency stash in the trash every couple of years. Better yet, give it away before it becomes worthless.

Small amounts of food additives aren't going to kill you, but don't live on foods laced with them. Use common sense. Stick to organic, natural foods as much as possible. The only problems you'll have with them are that they cost more and rot faster.

One of my favorite gripes related to toxins in food is the nasty way America treats chicken. In the late 1970s, as part of the "Let's Get Physical" craze, the nation arrived at the concept of "health food." And what made the list of health foods? Chicken and turkey.

America's poultry farmers had an immediate opportunity and a challenge. In 1975, the average person consumed about 26½ pounds of chicken and 6½ pounds of turkey. The craving for things with wings has gotten stronger every year since then.[1] Now chicken production—just chicken—is up to 500 million pounds a week. In twenty years Americans have doubled their chicken eating.

When you increase volume that dramatically in a business, you almost always see a decrease in quality. So it went in the world of chickens. In order to keep costs down while they increased output, chicken farmers added steroids to the grain. Then they dumped in antibiotics to keep the plumped-up chickens disease-resistant. Some of these foreign substances eventually made the hit list for government regulators, but not all. In short, unless you spend the money on free-range chicken, you may be feeding yourself and your kids the drugs of choice for chicken farmers. Needless to say, the same is true for turkeys. Three-pound birds waddling around the pen in August take up a big roasting pan by Thanksgiving, thanks to steroids.

Don't get me started on beef. Do you know how long it takes a cow that weighs eighty pounds at birth to get to a slaughter weight of about 1,400 pounds? A year to eighteen months. The time difference depends on how and what you feed her.

Think about how many times a week you ingest the growth tools of the chicken industry alone. Everything from your matzo ball soup to that pressed, preservative-laden lunchmeat called "98% fat-free sliced chicken breast" is putting trace amounts of hormones into your body.

Some physicians have a strong suspicion that this is a major contributing factor to the earlier onset of menstruation in American girls. Aside from high-hormone foods, high body fat in kids today is

---

[1] *The American Almanac: The Statistical Abstract of the United States,* 113th edition.

another suspected cause for early maturity. "That's life," you say. Well, Einstein, what about early menopause, which is the other side of the timeline?

I want you to challenge your eating habits not only to save yourself from disease and early death, but your family, too. Needless to say, you can't stop with waging a war on chicken. I've run into clients at the grocery store who have cheese curls and candy bars in the basket and they say, "That's for the children." A day or two later, they confess to me that they had a couple cheese curls. After they sweat through twenty-five push-ups, I say, "Who ate the rest of the bag?" "The kids," they say. "Thank you very much," I reply. "You are making darned sure I'm gonna be in business for at least another generation!"

What makes you think food that pollutes your body is okay for your kids? Because they "burn it off"? If they burn it off so well, why is one out of every five kids in the United States overweight or obese?[2] If it doesn't do any harm for our children to munch "fun" foods, why are about two-thirds of all teenage girls in the United States dysfunctional eaters?[3] The impact of bad eating, which includes not eating, goes far beyond appearance. Unhealthy eating causes serious diseases and disabling conditions, no matter how old you are.

Roll these words around your mouth, recruit: diabetes, hypertension, heart disease. They are directly linked to being overweight, as are some forms of cancer. Now ask yourself if you want one of these to shorten your kid's life. Oh yeah, don't even think about what they'll do to you.

If you're stuck on a desert island and you have to make a choice between eating healthy and exercising, eat healthy. Quality eating

[2] Shape Up America!, a campaign founded by Dr. C. Everett Koop, also gives us the shocking number that 58 million adult Americans—one-third of the adult population—are obese or overweight.

[3] According to Frances Berg, M.S., "Afraid to Eat: Children and Teens in Weight Crisis" (*Healthy Weight Journal*, 1997), more than half of fourteen-year-old girls in a study of 1,000 suburban Chicago girls had already been on one weight loss diet, approximately two-thirds of all teenage girls in the U.S. have abnormal eating behavior, and one-tenth of the teenage girls in the U.S. have potentially fatal eating disorders.

is about total health. Be emotional about your food by being passionate about eating right.

LISTEN UP!

To cut your craving for junk, make sure you're never hungry. Eat something good every couple of hours. And keep something decent in your car.

Eating out presents a special challenge if you're shy. The Sarge is not. I have no problem asking a restaurant to prepare food a particular way. Do I give a waiter a tip just to drop off a plate of noodles? Heck, no! If he wants his money, he can tell the chef that the sauce goes in a separate dish and I don't want cheese on my salad.

Some things are tough to do, like tell a chef he (or she) is doing his job wrong. Some things are really tough to do, like combining different types of food in the "ideal" way for the absorption of nutrients. Rather than plunge you into the science of sophisticated healthy eating, I'm keeping it simple.

SIMPLE CHANGES

Look at the palm of your hand. Now imagine a steak or burger sitting in it. Is it bigger than your hand? Yes? Then it's too big. If you can avoid the steroids and other junk I've already discussed, meat is not unhealthy for you if you go easy. In fact, it's the prime source of vitamin B12, so you have to be an extra intelligent eater if you abstain from meat. As a society, our problem with meat is just that we eat too much of it. The simple solution is never eat more meat in a day than you can fit in one hand. (That's *your* hand, jerky.) Notice I did not say that all the protein you eat in a day should fit in your hand—just meat.

On days when you decide you must have a cheeseburger, do yourself a favor and make it sort of healthy. Put it on a whole wheat or other whole grain bun instead of that worthless white stuff. And instead of iceberg lettuce, which is about as nutritious as a plastic bag, use a darker lettuce and slices of fresh tomato.

When you do cut back on meat, what do you put in that hole on your plate where the cow used to be? Beans. Does your family have a problem with eating beans when it's too cold to open the windows? Legumes are a good source of fiber, protein, and carbohydrates, and they give you the sensation of being filled up before you overload your body with calories.

One other thing: Eat your vegetables and fruits. They don't create miracles, so don't expect to jump through the roof because you ate a few carrots. You may notice small changes, though. If your gums bleed a little when you brush your teeth, you may find that adding a few more vitamins to your diet will stop that. And you just might feel more like pumping out a few extra push-ups. Hoooraahhh!

If you don't make all the changes in this chapter at once, fine. Start with one or two now and make them over time. It took me seven years to transform my eating habits. I have seen plenty of people make radical changes overnight, though, because they were scared. Maybe they had a heart attack or someone close to them had a heart attack—that will do it. Are you going to wait for that, or are you going to start now before you're scared?

For now, at least follow these three basic rules, and your honey will soon have to grab something besides love handles.

Rule Number One

Your meals should diminish in size as the day goes on. After all those exciting hours in the rack, you need to refuel before you start the day. Eating a big bowl of oatmeal in the morning makes as much sense as filling your gas tank before a long drive. Would you put a measly gallon of gas in the car if you were about to drive from Washington, D.C., to New York City? Would you drive the entire length of the New Jersey Turnpike hovering near "empty," then fill up when you arrived in The Bronx?

Rule Number Two

Don't overdo the carbohydrates—especially at night. Be careful about eating lots of carbohydrates before you go to bed. Your body breaks down carbohydrates into simple sugars and ultimately absorbs glucose into the bloodstream. Excess glucose is converted into glycogen, which is then stored around the body. You're supposed to use it up as energy, but guess what happens if you don't use up that energy snoring? Those extra carbohydrates can lead to an increase in body fat and more pounds. You want to stay away from things like bread and potatoes before bed, but an apple or glass of nonfat warm milk is fine. In fact, that milk may do more than just make you feel cozy: In order for your body to burn fat, *some* glucose has to be present in your system.

Rule Number Three

Eat roughly every two hours, starting when you get up. When your body is hungry, in order to keep going, it consumes muscle tissue. Muscle is the reason you're reading this book—you want it! If you have more active muscle tissue, you will have less fat. Metabolically active muscle tissue needs up to fifty calories a day per pound. You cannot gain muscle tissue if you starve yourself!

After you stop growing at about age twenty, unless you exercise and eat properly, you can lose up to one-half pound of muscle a year. That means by age forty, you need five hundred fewer calories a day if your activity level is the same and you don't eat to

Age 20 Profile: Male	Age 40 Profile: Male
5'9"	5'9"
Eats 3,500 calories a day	Eats 3,500 calories a day
Hangs around campus, plays pickup softball (everybody wants him on their team), does something active with his girlfriend daily	Hangs around the office, plays pickup softball (he's the outfield), does something mildly active with his wife once every three months
160-pound hunk	240-pound blob

Note: This problem applies to women, too, only worse.

maintain muscle. If you weigh more at age forty and have the same activity, you can bet your pension that extra weight is fat. At the rate of five hundred extra calories a day, you can put on ten, twenty, fifty pounds a year without doing anything different from year to year.

Women have a special challenge. Mother Nature knows that it takes about eighty thousand calories for a healthy baby to develop. That's twenty-four pounds, stored as fat, that Mother Nature wants you to keep as long as you have the potential to bear children. You starve yourself and she makes sure the weight loss doesn't reduce that "baby fat"; it comes from loss of muscle tissue. Female recruits, you do have it harder than men, but you're up to it!

Keep your metabolism high: Eat! Drink water! Kick butt!

SAMPLE MENU

I am going to assume that you are not a vegetarian, recruit. If I'm wrong, then hallelujah. Skip all the instructions on food that had a mother.

Breakfast

Big bowl of oatmeal or cereal: Look for natural ingredients, cereals low in preservatives that offer you more nutrients than refined sugar.

Low-fat or nonfat milk: Okay, so you're like most sane people who think that skim milk is really water with milk flavoring. Use the low-fat variety.

Fruit: What a treat. You get simple sugars with nutrients as a bonus.

Mid-morning snack

Half a whole wheat bagel, a banana, or real low-fat yogurt

I know you wouldn't make this mistake, but I've actually had recruits who thought that nonfat frozen yogurt was a healthy snack. If it's low in fat, it's high in something else to give it flavor. Like what? What did you promise to avoid during these three weeks? Sugar.

Lunch

Fruit

Sandwich: You thought I was going to slam raw vegetables down your throat, didn't you? Nope. Eating well is not supposed to be a torture. It is fine to put something that bled when it was alive between two pieces of decent bread and eat it. As much as possible, check the contents of the turkey or beef slices as well as the bread to keep the additives to a minimum.

Try something like this: turkey with mustard on whole wheat, rye, pumpernickel, or some other good bread; add lettuce, tomato, and pickles.

Watch your condiments. If you use mayonnaise and butter, think of spreading that fat on the inside of your blood vessels. Imagine it oozing through your body and ending up settling at your gut and butt. Hold that nightmare and let it force your hand to grab the mustard, lemon juice, or low-fat salad dressing instead. No condiments on a sandwich is always fine.

OR

Small salad: Again, watch what you put on it. I've seen plenty of fat people load up at the salad bar. Do they really think they're eating healthy by drowning helpless vegetables in a sea of blue cheese dressing? ("They" can easily be us. Personally, I love blue cheese dressing. It's tough for me not to abuse it. So who said this was always easy?)

Mid-Afternoon Snack

Fruit, a couple fig bars, a few rice cakes, air-popped popcorn, and a naked baked potato are examples of acceptable goodies. If you have something like rice cakes or a potato, you can expect an "energy spike." Go for a walk.

Late-Afternoon Snack

Eat something before you get home from work. Have a tall class of water; eat the other half of your whole wheat bagel. Keep supplies in your car: a bottle of water, a couple fig bars, a piece of fruit, an energy bar.

Dinner

Throw some shrimp or slices of grilled steroid-free animal on a big salad with low-fat dressing. For a treat, add a little avocado. Sure, it has fat, but it's the kind that's good for your cholesterol balance.

OR

Grill or bake a piece of fish and serve it with vegetables and a salad. Find ways to make it more exciting without fat. One way is adding a vegetable puree as a garnish.

Steam red peppers, then put them in the blender with a clove of garlic, salt, and pepper. If you use steamed carrots, add water, salt, and a little orange juice in the blender (fresh-squeezed, of course).

Nighttime Snack

Fruit is a good thing. This is the time of day when many recruits crave something sweet. Get your fix, but do it without involving fat. Stay away from the wicked desserts like ice cream and cheesecake. Just don't buy that stuff, and if you are not the food shopper in your house, put your foot down.

Anytime Snack

Before you shove something in your mouth ask yourself, "Did this grow out of the ground?" If the answer is yes, then you are in the category of "water-rich food." That's good, recruit. If you're hungry, eat it. The big exception is a white potato—that's a midday snack, not a late-night one. Most people aren't active enough at night to work off a potato. If you have an incredible sex life, I'll make an exception, but not every day.

Notice I did not give you portions. One reason is because all calories are not created equal. Right now, all I want you to do is clean up *what* you eat and you will see results. You can do it! You WILL do it!

CHAPTER FOUR
GET IN STEP, RICKY RECRUIT

Up in the mornin' with the risin' sun,
Crop-haired sergeant gonna make you run!

In Boot Camp, you will go for short humps (that means "jogs," civvies). So listen up 'cause I'm only going to say this once: *There are seven keys to getting it right.* If you get it right, you will have no pain and will lower your risk of injury. You will have sweaty clothes, a healthier body, a better attitude, hope for the future of mankind, and world peace. By the way, running and jogging are the same thing, and I'll use the terms interchangeably throughout the book. "Walking" is a different activity, described later in this chapter. Use it only if your nose will end up in the dirt if you jog.

In trying to adopt a good body position, use any reflective surfaces you pass—the windows of a building, for example. It isn't vanity, it's training. In preparing to earn my black belt in Hapkido, a martial art that literally means "the way (do) of power (ki) and coordination (hap)," I constantly used the mirrors in the dojo to refine my form. If you really have problems getting comfortable, ask a friend to videotape you running. You will be thrilled at the sight of your body in action because you will finally see where you must improve.

Memorize these seven keys!

1. Keep head up and eyes straight ahead.

Your chin should be parallel to the ground and your eyes focused in front of you. This does not mean your gaze should be so fixed that you lose sight of your environment. Don't be like Yeller.

Yeller the Mutt attended Boot Camp with his owner, Danny, who was one of my first clients and helped me get this program off the ground (thank you, Danny!). Yeller was low to the ground, solid, and fast. When the class would jog around a ball field, Yeller humped alongside with his ears flopping and his tongue hanging out. One morning, he tore around

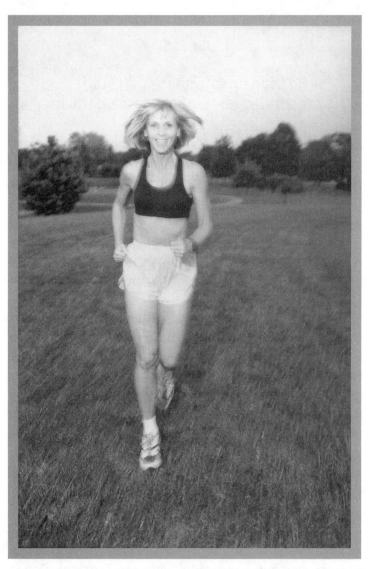

Head up, arms bent at the sides, breathin' easy, hair blowin' in the wind. It's always a good day to run if you know how.

the corner as usual and didn't notice that a net had been added to the soccer goal. Wham—right into the net! Arrgh, arrgh, arrgh.

Yeller did one thing right, though. As soon as he freed himself from the net, he got his legs in gear. Of course Danny and the rest of us laughed our heads off and Yeller was ready for more. If you get caught in a soccer net, or trip over a dead rock, don't get up and stare at the source of your embarrassment. Keep moving.

Don't bob your head, either. If you get tired and let your head wobble, you could get dizzy. The next thing you know, you'll have to stop jogging and start walking. Your objective is not to get dizzy and walk, it is to jog.

2. Hold shoulders erect, but relaxed.

A common mistake is slouching, or rolling the shoulders forward.

Run as if you're proud. The best way to do this is to imagine a string from the center of your chest or your bra with someone on the other end pulling you (don't get any crazy ideas, guys). There should be a slight arch in your back, but you should look like your chest is leading you.

3. Keep arms bent at a ninety-degree angle.

Imagine your arms are in a cast. Keep that basic position, but let your arms relax a little on the downswing. Don't hold them like a sprinter; they keep their arms very rigid. You're a jogger, so keep them fluid and loose. Reeeeeelax, reeeee-cruit.

4. Keep your wrists limp and let your thumbs slightly graze your sides as the arms swing downward.

Why do so many women run as if they're a Tyrannosaurus rex or Barney?

I think it's to hide the bouncing breasts. An iron jog bra should fix most of your bounce. Women, keep your hands where they belong. If you jog at a decent hour like 0600, no one will see you anyway except other recruits in your neighborhood.

Women and men, keep your wrists limp and let your thumbs brush your waistband. Your arms should be going back and

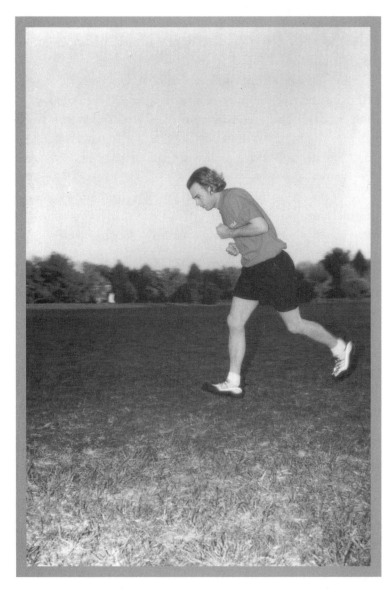

Straighten up! Stop looking for dog turds.

forth, perpendicular to your body, not rolling or crossing in front of you.

5. Foot strike is heel to toe.

If your foot hits toe to heel when you jog, you are running backward. We will not be running backward in Boot Camp.

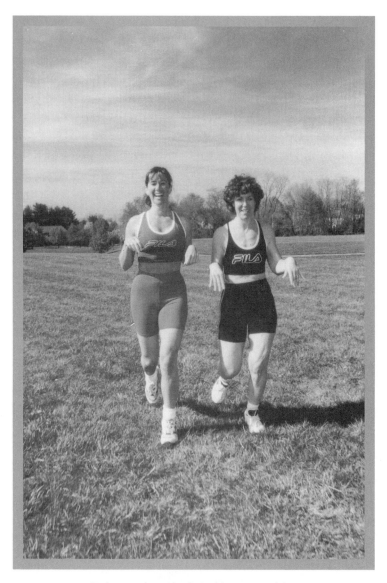

Put your hands down by your sides.
Who do you think you are—Barney?

Shuffle your feet; let them drag slightly on the ground until it's comfortable to pick them up higher. Just remember: You are not a horse, so no prancing.

Wear a running shoe, not a cross-trainer or tennis shoe.

Running shoes support a heel-to-toe motion: They have more cushioning in the heel than the toe. Throughout this entire program, wear new running shoes. That is an order. Period. They prevent your foot from rolling in (inversion) or out (eversion); they will help keep you off the injury list. I see plenty of folks who don't listen, and they end up injured.

6. Maintain an upright body position.

The muscles in your lower back are called erectors. (I once gave a lecture to a room full of women, and when explaining the erectors, the room went silent. It wasn't until later that day that I realized I had told them, "These are the muscles that keep me constantly erect.") Directly across from them on the front of your body, you have abdominal muscles. The job of abdominals is not just to make you look good in a bathing suit. Their main purpose is to work with the erectors to keep you upright. If they can't perform, your upper and lower body will form a ninety-degree angle and you will look like our ape ancestors. (Speaking of evolution, upright posture developed before large brains did.)[1]

7. Pace your breathing.

The most important thing about jogging is your breathing. If at any time your breathing gets ahead of you, that is, your breaths are racing but your body is not, slow down. That's an order! Should the problem become more severe and your breathing takes control of you, walk until you can breathe comfortably, then pick up the pace at a comfortable stride. As you master breathing and run greater and greater distances, you will find that the only part of you that gets tired when you run is your legs—never your lungs.

When you jog, take short breaths. Deep, or diaphragmatic, breathing is out in Boot Camp. Breathing during your run happens in four stages: in (first half of inhale), in (final half), out (first half of exhale), out (final half). That's in-in, out-out. As each foot hits the ground, you are at one stage or another in

---

[1] "The Dawn of Humans" series, *National Geographic*. (See, I do read!)

the series of four. These are small breaths, designed to keep you from constantly trying to catch your breath.

Breathe through your mouth. Your nose can be obstructed by boogers, sinus problems, your finger, or airborne insects. Your mouth should be slightly puckered, as if you were whistling.

Your buddy next to you should not be able to hear you breathing. Breathe lightly; take small breaths using the four count. You'll know you are jogging at the right intensity level if you can sing your favorite song from start to finish. If you have a hard time singing or talking—out loud, not in your head— you are going too fast. Is this understood? Good!

Stay very attentive to your breathing pattern for all thirty days. When you are done, who knows? You may even impress me (but don't count on it).

ASSIGNMENT ONE

Before you start jogging, go to a park or track where lots of people run and watch them. As the first twenty slog past you, notice what they are doing wrong and how many of them are doing things right. Record the results in your log.

Take special note of people who look comfortable, even happy, while they're running. Watch them breathe, examine their posture, check out that blissful look on their faces. Don't they make you feel like getting up and running with them?

ASSIGNMENT TWO

One day, pretend your car is broken. (Could this really happen?) Walk or jog where you have to go or hump to the nearest bus stop or train station.

I don't care if you do a fifteen-minute mile or a six-minute mile as long as your body position and breathing are right. The key to success is not how far you went, but how long you did it! There will be various times in this book when I will tell you to jog a specific distance, and that's to give you a goal. Nevertheless, the more important measure for Boot Camp is how many minutes you can jog, not what distance you went.

Now, listen up! Here are the Sarge's rules for jogging:

- During Boot Camp, don't use headphones. You need to get used to your jogging environment as well as the new stresses you are putting on your body. Wait until you are comfortable with the exercise to add music or world news.

- Don't jog at night. Ideally, do it first thing in the morning. There are two reasons for this. First is the safety issue associated with flaunting your little shorts in front of tired evening commuters and night crawlers. Second is the value of doing your entire Boot Camp regimen in the early morning. I want you to get in the habit of doing it at the same time every day, Monday through Friday. For most people, it is much harder to adhere to a schedule like that at night.

- Regardless of the brand, if your running shoes are more than six months old, get a new pair. Even if you never used them and they are still sitting in the original box, if your shoes are six months old, they are garbage. There is cheap cushioning in the heels of the shoes that is not designed for longevity. If you run with old or inferior shoes, you will get hurt. Save them for mowing the grass or give them to somebody with no shoes.

- Dress for your climate. Go to a running store (not some cheesy department store) where people theoretically know what the ideal fabrics are for the weather in your area. You don't have to spend a lot of money; you are interested in fabric, not fashion. For example, cotton feels good as you begin your run, but it quickly loses its appeal when you sweat because it dries slowly. Jog bras with a nylon-polyester-spandex combination and 100 percent nylon shorts offer greater comfort than cotton. Beware of wearing too much clothing. If you perspire and a layer of wet clothing sticks to your body, you will get cold and develop a dreadful attitude. Finally, if it's raining, wear a hat. Hooghraah!

- Take a water bottle with you if you are going to be jogging fifteen minutes or more. At the running store, you can buy a belt that encircles your hips and holds a small water bottle store (or you can call me and order an official Boot Camp Belt). Don't cheat on this, recruit! Water lubricates your joints and maintains your body's temperature. Without sufficient water, you will feel dizzy and fatigued. Some people suffer from headaches and irritability without enough water.

- Before jogging, always void your body of any substance that may want to leave you. When you're jogging, if something wants to leave, it will leave. You don't want to be in some nice neighborhood and get caught using the admiral's bushes. And don't drink coffee or eat a lot before you run. If you eat too much before you jog, you will go to the bathroom before you finish. I don't want my recruits to soil their communities.

- Try to run on blacktop or a track (yawn) rather than concrete or a field. Concrete is hard on your joints; an open field can contain surprises like divots and dog crap. The downside of a track is that the scenery doesn't change no matter how many times you circle it. If you do use a track, run in the outside lane and switch directions every other lap. This will help you avoid stressing the same muscles every time. If you jog the quarter-mile circumference of a football field during Boot Camp, round the corners to save your ankles. Wherever you do decide to run, make sure it's flat, not hilly. Jogging up and down hills can cause cramps and shinsplints. Oh, and make sure you like being wherever you run since you're going to be there for quite a while.

- If you get an abdominal cramp and jogging hurts, walk until it dissipates. Try rubbing the area—it's usually near the lower part of your rib cage—to stimulate blood flow, since this cramp is generally caused by lack of blood flow to the respiratory muscles.

- If your knees, ankles, or back hurt, walk. "Hurt" doesn't mean "feel(s) tired," so stay honest. Often the new Boot Camp trainees who have pain in those areas need to lose weight. Is that you, recruit? If so, take off some fat before you graduate from a walk to a jog. Another common cause of joint pain is bad shoes. Go shopping. Another possible cause is that your muscles don't have enough conditioning to take the load. In that case, wait until you're stronger before you jog. Listen to your body, and don't push yourself into the realm of pain. If you damage yourself, you will crush your spirit, then this book will sit on your shelf collecting dust. That will make me very mad, young soldier.

- Don't sprint the last part of your jog. It's an explosive exercise that could easily damage your muscle tissue and the benefits are nil. It's something foolish you did in high school, and when I say, "Be all you used to be," I don't mean be as foolish as you used to be.

> Chuck wouldn't listen that morning. Sergeant Lawrence told him to take it slow and cool down, but he decided to sprint to the finish. When the group caught up, they saw him in someone's yard across the street. That day he had a black hat and black T-shirt, so in the predawn light Chuck looked like a hoodlum. "Get out of there, man," Sergeant Lawrence yelled, "or somebody's going to think you're here to rob him." Chuck didn't listen. He just stood there in the yard with his hands on his hips as his head was hanging down. As the sergeant came closer, he noticed Chuck's face matched the grass. That morning, his name changed to "Up-chuck."

Within thirty days, 60 percent of the people I see become addicted to jogging, and there are two reasons why. First, it is usually the exercise that is the easiest when it's done correctly. Second, you notice, and feel, rapid progress, so it gives you a sense of accomplishment. Stay comfortable as you learn to jog and you will probably be one of the addicts. Photocopy the checklist below and take it with you to help you improve as you go through Boot Camp. If your progress doesn't meet your expectations, log on to the web site and ask some questions. I'll tell you in advance that the reason most people will ask for help is because they forgot what I said about breathing. YOU won't forget anything I say, will you, recruit?

Due to circumstances beyond your immediate control, if you *cannot* jog, become a walker, swimmer, or biker. If you must be indoors because you live in the upper peninsula of Michigan (yaaah aaaye) and it's colder than a witch's navel (brrr), then walk up and down stairs slowly for twenty minutes. Whatever you do, do it continually, then move straight to your other Boot Camp exercises.

1. Keep head up and eyes straight ahead.

2. Hold shoulders erect, but relaxed.

3. Keep arms bent at a ninety-degree angle.

4. Keep your wrists limp and let your thumbs slightly graze your sides as the arms swing downward.

5. Foot strike is heel to toe.

6. Maintain an upright body position.

7. Pace your breathing (1-2, 3-4; in-in, out-out).

8. Keep water in your body.

You've been walking ever since you found out how to balance your diapered butt over your chubby little legs, but I'll bet you don't know how to walk for exercise. Muggers (that's right, I mean bad guys) love the way most people walk—slow pace, drooping upper bodies, and a bored look on their faces. Change all that. Scare the muggers away with your determined look, confident stride, and quick step. Remember the seven keys to jogging correctly? The keys to power walking are similar, but pay attention: They are not identical.

1. Keep head up and eyes straight ahead.

You already know you need to lift your head, but don't go to extremes. Some people think "hold your head high" means "look like a snob." Keep your chin at a normal level.

2. Hold shoulders erect, but relaxed.

In walking, you will have one small movement that you don't in running. Because you are swinging your arms, your shoulders will rotate slightly. Don't force them, though, or you will look goofy.

3. Keep arms bent at slightly less than a ninety-degree angle.

Keep arms fluid and loose while they enjoy a natural swing that picks up the determination on your face. On the upswing, don't slam your arm through the air as if you're looking for a fight. On the downswing, make sure your arm goes no further than your running shorts.

4. Thumbs should slightly graze your sides as the arms swing downward.

Not only will this keep you from looking like T-Rex with your hands dangling at your chest, but it will prevent you from making a fist with your hands. Clenched hands feed tension to your entire body.

5. Foot strike is heel to toe.

Again, you want to walk forward, so go heel to toe. Try a move that walking coach Elaine Ward calls "rolling footwork."[2] Keep your feet low to the ground as you would with a jog, but roll one foot from heel to toe, then the next, giving yourself a slight push forward with your back toe.

If you naturally walk like a duck or a pigeon, practice walking straight. That's right, I said "practice." Forcing yourself to go from years of waddling to hours of walking straight could actually hurt you. Retrain yourself gradually.

Some shoe companies make special models for walking, but go ahead and invest in running shoes for a couple of good reasons. First, running shoes support the heel-to-toe motion that is essential in both jogging and running, and second, the idea in Boot Camp is to walk briskly only when you cannot jog. You will graduate to a faster pace very shortly, recruit, and you will need those running shoes.

6. Hip and leg action is smooth and tight.

Take a look at people on the sidewalk. Watch how many swing their butts as if they want to bump everyone else into the gutter. Their lower back and hips are building up a lot of resentment. You, on the other hand, will build endurance.

As you walk erectly on your mile-long path, take short, quick steps and move your hip with your leg. After all, the two are connected. If you do this correctly, your feet will not be far apart from each other. In fact, it may look as if they're landing almost in front of each another.

7. Pace your breathing.

Breathing during your walk happens in four stages. Each

2 Elaine P. Ward, *Walking Wisdom for Women* (Acumen Technologies, 1995).

time you step, you take a quarter breath—two steps are in-in, and two steps are out-out.

If you're already throwing money at a health club, go there and practice walking on the treadmill near a mirror. Watch your form and check your breathing. I don't recommend this for jogging, because it's too easy to fall off.

On days when you're bored with walking and ready for more fun, do what I did with my first client, a diplomat who paid me to come to his house and train him first thing in the morning. Three times a week, we'd walk the streets near his house. As we would go through a park in his neighborhood, I'd make him climb a fence that was in our way. This wasn't easy for a forty-year-old fat man who went everywhere in a chauffeured limousine, but he laughed all the way through it. He thought I was cuckoo. Can you imagine that?

CHAPTER FIVE
SPREAD 'EM

STOP KVETCHING AND START STRETCHING!

In Boot Camp, you will be sore. Do you want to be stiff, too? Let me fill you in on stiff. Stiff is walking around as if you've just gotten off a horse after a five-hour ride and you have a bad case of inflamed hemorrhoids. OUCH! Sound like fun? Well unless you stretch your muscles after using them, you will not only be sore, but you will be stiffer than a Cowboy who just lost to the Redskins (go 'Skins). Whether you are contracting your muscles through exercise or everyday activities, lengthen them again or your body will get rigid; life will become one uncomfortable moment after another. Why do you have to stretch your neck? Because you spend endless hours a day with your head locked onto computers, TVs, and oncoming traffic. Why do a butt stretch? Because you sit on your butt most of the time.

I ran my first marathon (26.2 miles) in October 1992, and for days I couldn't sit on the can, let alone walk down a flight of stairs without looking like I had a potato chip in my butt that wouldn't break! I was sooo darn tired after the race that all I wanted to do was sleep, not stretch. I learned my lesson and I'm sharing it: Stretch, soldier, stretch.

My definition of aging is lack of flexibility. If it hurts to move, you won't move. You'll start to annoy your kids and your spouse, and the next thing you know you will be a lazy bum asking others to do every little task. Are you laughing? Are you thinking, "*I* won't do that." Bull! Just look around you. What are your mom and dad like? How about your friends? Do you, or they, have anyone helping with ordinary activities around the house and yard—waxing a floor, painting a fence, raking leaves? These things don't require strength. You need flexibility and a little bit of endurance.

We get busy in our world of specialization, doing only what we get paid for and saving the rest for teenagers who will shovel snow for ten bucks or college kids who will wash our windows for fifty dollars. Get off your lazy behind and do it yourself! The best thing you could do for yourself is to do something by yourself. Paint your own house, mow your own grass, chop that tree down with your own two hands, and use every one of those chores as an opportunity to stretch. Pick up a tool and get moving, but first, listen to this important message.

My brother Richard owns a construction business in Florida, and he is always complaining that his back is sore. Let's think about that for a minute. He is in construction, so the odds are high that his back and stomach muscles get a lot of use. He is constantly lifting himself and heavy objects, so he's strong, right? Actually, he is strong as an ox, so what's missing? Two things, but stretching is the main one. When he gets home, he hits the La-Z-Boy, grabs a cold beer, and lights the fire of the big screen. He works his butt off, so I don't blame him, but that's not what he should do. He should stretch for about ten minutes before he plops in the chair and ten minutes in the morning before he goes to work. (I can see him laughing as he reads this.) The second thing he should do, of course, is pay attention to *how* he lifts himself and his tools. Does he listen to me? It's hard to be a prophet in your own village.

Assignment One

Here is a real eye opener. (By the way, I did this as well as every other exercise in this book. How else do you think I know they work so well?) If you want a real incentive to stretch, go to a nursing home. Sit in the lobby for ten minutes and imagine you live there. Imagine what it's like to know the smallest movement will break you in half, and how humiliating it is to ask for help to zip your pants or button your dress. Record your observations and feelings in your log.

By the way, *USA Today* published results of a 1997 survey funded by the National Institute on Aging that indicated many women ages forty to fifty-five have problems related to weakness and decreased flexibility. Twenty percent of those surveyed have trouble climbing stairs, carrying groceries, even dressing or bathing themselves. Fifty-five percent suffer from stiffness or soreness in their joints, neck, or shoulders. What is going on here? These women should be in their prime and they can't even snap their own bras without a struggle. The article pointed out it's "mostly a matter of whether you exercise and what you eat. As it is for most men and women of all ages."[1] Got that guys? The warning applies to you, too, even though you escaped this particular study.

Who is confined to a nursing home? People who cannot (due to injury or disease) or have refused to (due to laziness) move their bodies. They can't bend over to tie their own shoe laces. Shoe laces, heck! They can't bend over to pet the dog, or get dressed, or even eat without assistance. Please don't get me wrong, now: I mean no disrespect for the elderly and sick. I am specifically pinpointing the folks who have done nothing to help themselves stay limber. (In the

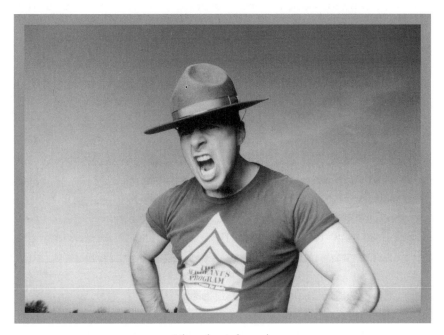

Nice dental work.

[1] Al Neuharth, "How midlife women can cure most hurts," *USA Today*, October 17, 1997, 13A.

next chapter, I'll tell you about the impact of strength training on elderly people.)

Condition your body for life's daily tasks, starting now! Think of the people who can't tie their shoes and yell, "That's NOT what I want to be, Sarge!"

Don't let bad habits and a bad attitude put you in a wheelchair at a time in your life when you could be playing with your grandchildren or walking down a shaded lane with your sweetheart. When you stop moving your body, that's when you start to die.

Some day, you want to be an elderly person with a young and spirited attitude and a body that can still perform efficiently (even with the lights on). As long as you use this book, recruit, that's the kind of person you are destined to become.

Bill Mohan, a six-year veteran of our early morning abuse, and I went on a twenty-mile run one day, and he told me a story so profound I felt you should hear it. Bill's elderly dad was supposed to visit the family for the Christmas holidays, so Bill drove over to the retirement home to pick him up. Good ol' Dad had his bags packed and was ready to go with only one minor problem. Walking had become too "difficult" for him, so he had treated himself to a wheelchair. Bill was frustrated, to say the least, when he saw his dad sitting comfortably in that chair. Of course he would be—Bill is a forty-five-year-old maniac who runs 'til his feet fall off. So Bill said, "No way, Pops. No wheelchair, but I will make you a deal: For your two-week visit, I will walk with you every day up and down the street, and when you are tired we will rest." The elderly Mr. M. said, "Okay, I'll try it." So they did. The evening after he returned to his retirement home, he called Bill and thanked him, saying, "I can walk to the chow hall!" Way to go, Bill! By the way, Bill's dad never used a wheelchair again in all the years he lived after that Christmas.

Now get off your butt and let's get started! Stretching should be done when your muscles are warm. Should you stretch before your daily run? Yep, but only after you warm up. Remember how to do that, recruit? Walk your dog or do some other mild exercise for five minutes. It's okay if it's fun. Should you stretch after your run? Yep. Some people don't need to stretch much; they're naturally flexible. Trust me, if you're reading this book, that's not you.

Here are the Sarge's rules on stretching:

1. Do it when you're warm and do it between exercises.

You are warm if you have some perspiration on your forehead from movement or you have been briskly moving for a minimum of five to eight minutes.

You are also warm, I hope, if you're taking a shower or soaking in a bubble bath. Doing gentle stretches after you get out of the shower or while you play with your duckie in the tub is fine. (I play with my battleship.)

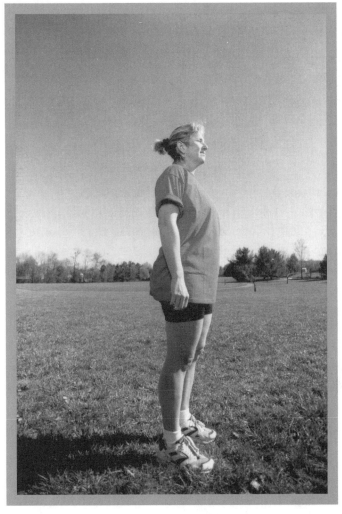

Whether your stretch involves a standing or sitting

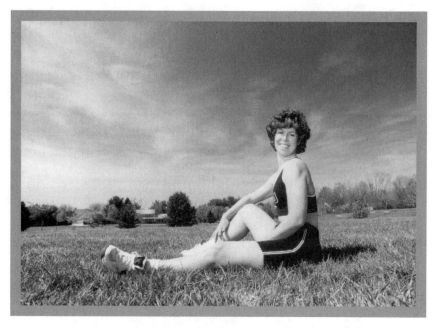

position, start with a straight back.

2. As long as you're in Boot Camp, stretch twice a day.

If you do Boot Camp workouts in the morning, stretch again every night before Mommy tucks you in. If you do your Boot Camp workout in the evening, then do your second set of stretches in the morning *after* you warm up. To warm up, you can walk up and down your stairs ten times, briskly walk a constipated dog, or have a romp with your spouse.

3. Keep your body in perfect alignment.

For most stretches, think of your body as a robot, moving cleanly on an axis—up and down, side to side, in and out. When you're in alignment, you have the muscles in the ideal position to stretch. The stretch is a lot easier on you and will be done effectively. It will help you visualize and achieve the proper alignment if you keep in mind that a muscle is attached on two different bones, otherwise it wouldn't be a proper lever.

4. Hold the stretch for a few seconds, relax, then repeat that stretch several times.

While holding the stretch, the objective is to relax the muscle that you are trying to stretch. Only when the muscle is relaxed, can you stretch it properly. If you do it with force, it will tighten. There is a "sensor" within the muscle that tells it to tighten or relax; you have to do what it takes to get it to relax. If you are trying to do a hamstrings stretch, for example, keep your back straight and torso in alignment. Contract the thigh muscles (quadriceps), which are the *opposing* muscles to the hamstrings, while you lean forward. Lean forward until you feel a slight tightness in the hamstrings, hold for a few seconds, then relax. The following chart indicates which muscle groups you tighten, or contract, and which ones you relax in the particular "active isolated stretch" (AIS):

Stretch	Muscle Tightened	Muscle Relaxed
hamstrings	quadriceps	hamstrings
thighs	hamstrings	quadriceps
lower back	abdominals	erectors
chest	upper back	pectorals
calves	shin muscle	calves
butt	hip flexor	gluteus maximus

5. Don't do "bounce stretching," also known as "ballistic stretching."

There are dozens of stretching techniques promoted by trainers for people at different fitness levels, and bouncing is not the one for you. In Boot Camp, you will stretch slowly, with no radical moves. Ballistic stretching is known to make you sensitive to injury, possibly tearing muscle fibers. That will create problems for you now and down the road.

You won't catch every muscle every time you stretch, but you should always work the big ones: hamstrings (back of the legs), quadriceps (thighs), gluteus maximus (butt), erectors (lower back), pectorals (chest), and deltoids (shoulders).

Sit down and get ready to work!

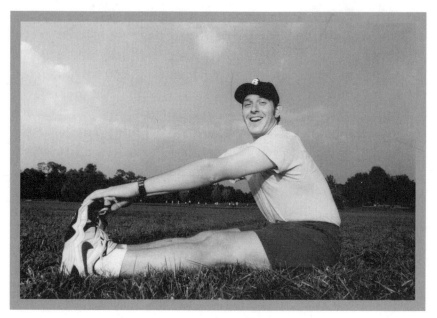

Reach, but don't pull or bounce. And let me see you smile.

LISTEN UP!

When I tell you to hold a stretch, I mean hold it for a solid ten seconds. That's "one thousand and oooonnnne, one thousand and twoooooooo, one thousand and threeeeeeeee . . ."

Hamstrings Stretch

Remember that stupid exercise called a cherry picker? You know, you were in high school and your gym teacher barked, "Stand up straight! Now touch your toes! Again! Again!" Don't EVER do that again. Sarge has a much safer way to stretch your hamstrings—one that won't send your back into spasms.

Sit down with your legs in front of you. Toes together pointed straight up in the air. Almost lock your legs, so your knees are flat on the ground. With your back *straight* and your chest sticking out, reach forward toward your knees. If you touch your knees, go for your

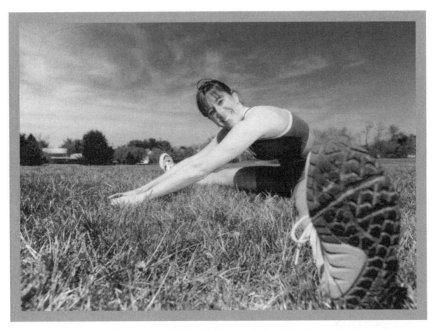

If you could do this, you'd smile, too.

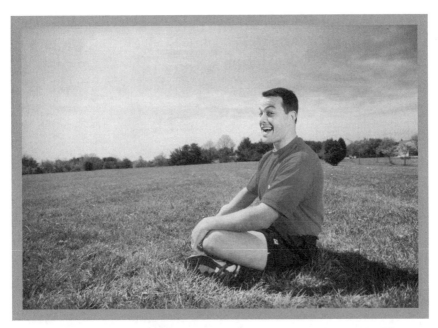

A silly grin won't stretch your lower back. Lean forward with
your head down.

shins. If you get your shins, try your ankles. If you get your ankles, go for your socks. If you get your socks, go to your toes. Just make sure that whatever you touch belongs to you. Hold it—don't bounce.

Straddle Stretch

Still sitting with legs in front of you? Good—spread 'em! Toes still pointed in the air. Reach forward as far as you can in between.

You might try "walking" your hands forward on your fingertips to increase the stretch—just don't overdo it. I don't want your head getting stuck between your thighs.

Lower Back Stretch

Cross your legs "Indian style" or at least get as close as you can comfortably. Arch your back, lean forward, and drop your head down.

The Sergeant's Salute

Here's where you get to show me how you really feel about me.

Lie on your back. Spread your legs a little and pull your knees

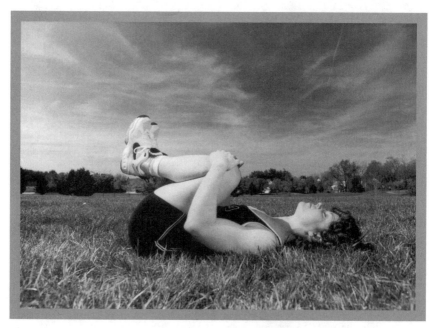

A real Sergeant's Salute is reeeeelaxing.

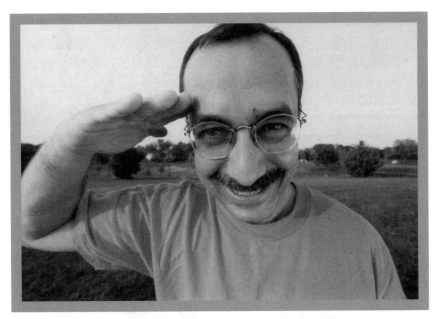

Only the buttnuts salute me this way.

into your chest. This is the same position you used as a kid when you yelled "Cannonball" and jumped into the pool. Your butt goes in the air facing me (hence the name "The Sergeant's Salute"). Hold that for ten seconds and stretch your gluteus to the max-imus.

Quad Stretch

Stand up. Find your partner. If you don't have a partner, find someone to put your arm around. (Stand by for other instructions if you hate to touch people.) Grab a thigh, preferably your own. With your knees next to your partner's, press forward with the pelvis, then pull one leg back by grabbing the ankle.

You should do this with your free hand. Use your partner to hold you up, and vise versa. Don't forget to stretch your other leg, too.

You can also try this without grabbing anyone or anything, but you might lose your balance. If that happens, pinch your earlobe

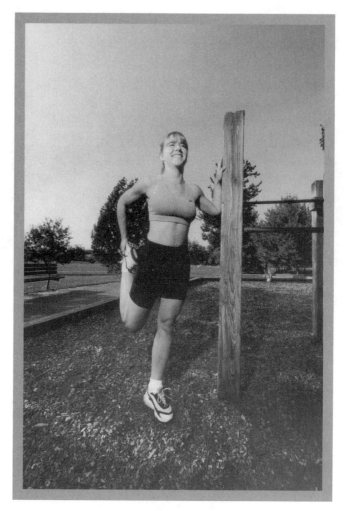

This is more fun with a partner than a pole, but you take what you can get.

with your free hand. Don't laugh, it works. The alternative is to grab a pole, door frame, or the handle on your car door.

POW Stretch

Remain standing. Put your fingertips together behind your head, with your elbows out. Think of the enemy surrendering. This will feel as if you're trying to crush a walnut with your shoulder blades.

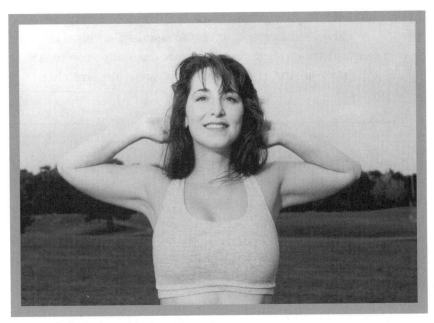

After push-ups, you'll want to surrender.

Arm Circles and Finger Crunches

Still standing, stick your arms out and rotate them. While rotating them, wiggle your fingers as if you're playing the piano, then close your hands in a fist. Imagine yourself squeezing a sponge or a ball. Make your circles bigger and bigger, but as the rotations get larger, bend your elbows more. Do this in counts of ten.

Shrugs

Let your hands rest on the quadriceps and elevate your shoulders toward your ears. Roll them slowly and do ten in each direction.

Neck Stretch

Eyes right, hold for ten. Don't forget to move your head with your eyes. Eyes left, hold for ten. Drop your chin(s) on your chest. Don't get radical with this stretch: We do NOT do neck circles in Boot Camp, just small turns and tilts. Too much head turning can be hard on your vertebrae, so don't twist your head like you're possessed.

Fitness comes in three parts, recruits. Remember your entrance exam? I checked your aerobic, or cardiovascular, endurance; your muscle endurance, or strength; and your flexibility. You're not fit unless you have all three, so don't blow past the stretches and cheat yourself!

CHAPTER SIX
MOVE YOUR BUTT

You think this is fun, don't you? Now, this is where the boot meets the butt—exercise!

In this chapter of your life, you will learn the proper way to do push-ups, dips, crunches, pull-ups, and the superman. That's it— that's all you need. You don't have to do them yet, though. Heck no! Why would you pay close attention to my instructions, then feel compelled to get on the floor and actually try to do these exercises correctly? Because I'm the Sarge and I told you to, that's why, you worthless bag of atrophy! Now listen up!

Need better reasons? Okay. Sargie has science to back him up. In one study,[1] seventy-two people in a weight-loss program followed the same diet, but not the same exercise regimen. Twenty-two of them did nothing except thirty-minute cardio workouts three days a week for eight weeks. Those fat-burners dropped an average of three pounds of lard in that time, but they also lost half a pound of muscle. The other fifty also worked out three times a week, but they did fifteen minutes of aerobic exercise and fifteen minutes of strength training. Sounds more like Boot Camp, doesn't it? These lucky people lost an average of ten pounds of fat and gained two pounds of muscle in the same eight weeks. Since muscle is like the chassis of your body—without it you don't have much shape—who do you think looked better after the experiment was over?

Let me tell you another story that will make you itch to do your strength exercises. (If you itch from exercise, that's your fault.) In

[1] Wayne L. Westcott, Ph.D., "Slowing Down the Clock," *Cycling & Fitness*, vol. 1, no. 2, 1990, 13–15.

1988, Dr. Maria Fiatarone at Tufts University Nutrition Center for Research in Aging did a reconditioning study with residents of the Hebrew Rehabilitation Center for the Aged. These men and women who were in the neighborhood of ninety years old were not paralyzed, but needed a walker, cane, or wheelchair to move around. Dr. Fiatarone wanted to see if resistance training could increase their muscle strength enough so they could walk without assistance. For eight weeks, they used their body weight and light weights three times a week to condition their quads and hips. In other words, the only exercises they did were a few for their legs and butts—that's it. Guess what? Of the nine people who completed the training, every one of them improved. Every single one of them had let their muscles atrophy so much that they needed assistance to do the most basic of exercises—walk.

Some people in this study graduated from the chair to a cane; others walked unassisted. Most graduated to their legs and were able to walk with no help at all. Can you imagine that—yes! Can you imagine the opposite—being so poorly energized that they had to sit all the time, letting their muscles atrophy so completely that they couldn't even walk to the bathroom to use the mirror to pick that booger that's been hanging out of their hairy nostrils for the last hour? Their dignity, their sense of self-esteem had to be in the basement because they caused the problem themselves.

When the study ended, what do you think happened? They reverted! Go figure. I guess everyone needs a drill instructor.

Dr. Fiatarone came back the following January, and this time she brought a total of one hundred patients into the study, including those who had participated the first time. Four years later, she was still getting the same results—every single patient had a noticeable increase in functional strength.[2] By the time the study ended,

---

[2] Dr. Fiatarone (and coauthors) documented the results of her initial study entitled "High-Intensity Strength Training in Nonagenarians (Effects on Skeletal Muscle)" in the *Journal of the American Medical Association,* June 13, 1990, vol. 263, no. 22. Her larger study including 100 elderly patients was documented in "Exercise Training and Nutritional Supplementation for Physical Frailty in Very Elderly People," published in *The New England Journal of Medicine,* June 23, 1994, 330:1769–1775.

her oldest participant was one hundred years old. Now, if you haven't just clutched this book to your breast and screamed, "Hallelujahhh! I looooove exercise, Sarge!" what are you waiting for, soldier?

Got the point, recruit? Human beings *need* to do strength conditioning in order to remain mobile. You will see this again, so heads up. Our bodies were designed for hard work, not sitting on our cans all day staring at screens. That's why we need resistance training. We have no choice, so we might as well make it fun!

The exercises in this chapter will counter the atrophy that comes from a life in which your ass spends hours a day in a chair. I will get you used to placing a load on your body. Building muscle tissue—hypertrophy—is the point of all these exercises. Even though you may not want to become more muscular, you do want the muscle you have to be stronger, metabolically active, and to replace some of the tissue you've lost over the years. Remember back in chapter 3 when I told you how much muscle tissue you can lose each year? Good! (If your memory is like mine, you need help: The answer is half a pound if you do nothing to retain it.) We're trying to stop that loss and even put on a few extra pounds of lean muscle tissue. And don't worry. You will not be a muscle freak like the folks on late-night ESPN. To look that way you need to eat about six thousand calories per day, have incredible genetics, lift weights a couple hours every day, and take

I had just finished teaching class one morning and a client named Big Talkin' Jay yelled to me that he had to leave. He was going to follow another client named Liz to a gas station so she could get the flat tire fixed on her Lexus. I made her change her own tire. She was forty-eight years old and had no idea how to change a tire. Not only did I save her from trashing her rim by driving on a flat to the gas station, but I gave her some bonus exercise and a new skill. What a guy!

steroids. So don't flatter yourself and relax. You'll end up looking normal.

Anytime you don't feel like doing these exercises, close your eyes and picture yourself as frail and bedridden. You're thinking, "I'm not even close to that." Tomorrow comes steadily, one day and step at a time. First, you have someone shovel snow for you, then you call a tow truck instead of changing your own flat tire. Pretty soon, you're afraid to haul your own trash. At some point you *can't* do it. Don't think that I have a deranged imagination, because I see it every day.

Our office for Boot Camp is on the second floor of a building, and I get complaints from lots of new Boots that they have to come up a flight of stairs to register for the program. That's one flight of stairs! I'll tell you what I tell them: I will get your behind in crack shape *if* you just care. Just take the time. Say out loud right now, "I CAN-NOT LIVE THIS WAY! I MUST CHANGE!" If you say that and mean it, you can win. I am 100 percent serious! Otherwise pass this book on to someone else.

If you're still reading this book, that means you care. It means you can drag your big butt and gut over to me, look me in the eye-balls, and say, "Hey, man, I am sick and tired of being tired and sick and must make changes."

Hooraghhhhhh! Drop and give me ten! And if you can't give me ten yet, try one. If you can't do that, screw it. Just drop.

BUILDING STRENGTH

Push-ups

(My personal favorite exercise—and soon to be yours—to which I attribute my sense of humor.)

Upper body strength means that you can carry everything from groceries to babies to stacks of this book for your friends. You will be ready for everything from intramarital communication (other-wise known as doing the wild thing or mogombu-mumbo) to soft-ball at the company picnic.

Start by kneeling on the floor. Place your hands a little bit more

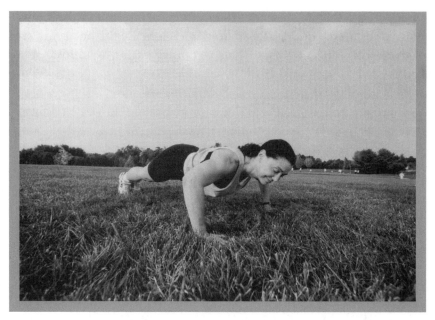

Her form is just as good on number 25.

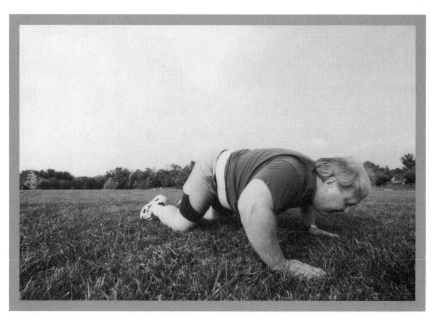

Just started Boot Camp and he's on his way to being all he used to be
in the Navy.

than shoulder width apart; point fingers straight ahead. Position your hands under the shoulder region. Begin by trying this exercise on your toes with legs extended—the "standard push-up."

Your body is straight as you do a standard push-up. In order to accomplish this, you actually have to raise the buttocks slightly. (That's *slightly.* No air humping!) Three points on your body come toward the ground simultaneously: nose, nipples, and navel. If these have lowered over the years, pretend you are twenty years old again.

Do the "modified push-up" with your knees on the ground if one of the following applies:

A competitive adventure racer, a woman who climbs mountains; swims through icy, raging waters; rides a mud-caked bike through the woods; and camps with bears and snakes for days at a time, came to my "ladies' butt-smokin', take-no-prisoners" class. I yelled, "Drop and give me twenty-five." All the women, lined up precisely in a row, delivered twenty-five push-ups instantly. They stretched and did some more. Then they stretched and did some more. Finally, I said, "Give me as many push-ups as you can."

The guest athlete assumed the standard position once again and resumed the exercise. I noticed her looking tired. She shot a glance to her left, then to her right. The heads on either side of her were going up and down, up and down. Finally, she collapsed and I laughed at her. She got huffy and said, "Don't laugh at me! This is embarrassing! I'm supposed to be an elite (ego) athlete!" Eventually, she found out the other women had dropped to their knees after the first set. (P.S. This competitive wingnut racer is Maryann, my coauthor.)

- A standard push-up makes you puke.
- You are pregnant.
- You have not done a push-up in fifty years and your arms feel like stale carrots.
- You have done a bunch of standard push-ups and you need to move to a modified push-up to do the exercise properly.

In the modified push-up, keep your back straight. Be sure to cross the ankles and bring the heels into the butt. This keeps your body weight off your kneecaps and shifts it to your thighs. Looks like you're doing a standard push-up. In fact, if someone saw just your upper body, that person would think you're on your toes, not your knees.

As a last resort, if you do not have the upper body strength to do even a modified push-up, do it against the wall as described in chapter 1.

Dips

(To get rid of your "bingo" arms.)

Have you ever noticed when you're waving good-bye to someone, your arm keeps waving after you've stopped? Or that your granny has that big flab of fat on the back of her arms? Those are "bingo" arms. Nasty, yes? Deep underneath that hunk of flab, way below those years of indulgence and atrophy are your triceps. You are about to transform that saggy, three-headed muscle into a source of power and pride. You are about to take this pendulous flap of adipose tissue and turn it into a smooookin' stack of muscle!

What is it good for?

Lowering your ass onto the toilet seat
Lowering yourself onto your chair
Pushing yourself into/out of your car
Washing your hair

Find a park bench, kick the drunk off, and use his shoe to clean off the bird crap. You can also use any level, solid surface that is

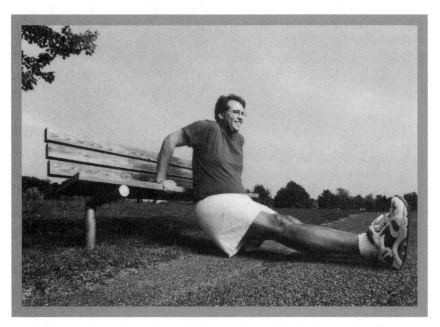

Bend your knees if the straight-legged position is impossible for you.

about two feet high, with or without bird crap. Scoot your butt to the edge of the bench. Put your hands over the edge of the bench with your fingers pointed forward and your thumbs under your butt. Put your feet out in front of you with your knees slightly bent.

With your arms holding you steady, lift off, bending your arms, so you can feel the back of your butt and your back grazing the bench. (If you don't bend your arms, you are doing an air hump.) Go down a little bit and come up. You should feel this in the back of your arms. If you don't, you're doing it wrong. One repetition is one dip.

Crunches

(Tight guts drive me nuts!)

Posture—that's really why we do crunches. You can pretend you do them to look like a pretty boy on the cover of a men's fitness magazine or a contestant for Miss Life Quest. The reality, though, is that you have to do them because you will slump over like an ape if

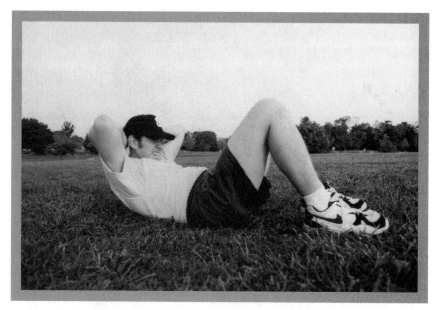

The dorks who do crunches this way must think they're a neck exercise.

you don't. Your abdominal muscles keep you erect. You must strengthen your abdominal muscles and erectors to walk like a proper Homo sapiens. (Stay tuned for the superman, which works your erectors.)

Most folks like to do abdominal crunches with their hands placed behind their neck. I do not want you pulling your head to your chest instead of using your abdominals to raise your head off the floor, so begin this way:

Fold your arms across your chest. Let your neck have some responsibility for controlling that thirteen-pound bucket you call a head. Bend your legs and plant your feet firmly on the ground, shoulder-width apart. This position takes the lower back out of the exercise. Using your abdominals, lift your upper back off the ground.

For most people, that will be where your bra back ends. Men, you know where that is. Lower yourself back down to the ground. Whenever you come up, squeeze the abdominals.

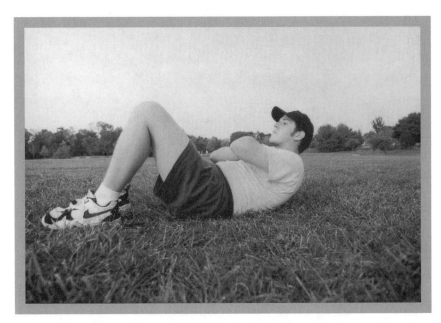

Start out in this position, and raise up until your bra strap is off the ground. If you don't have a bra, borrow one.

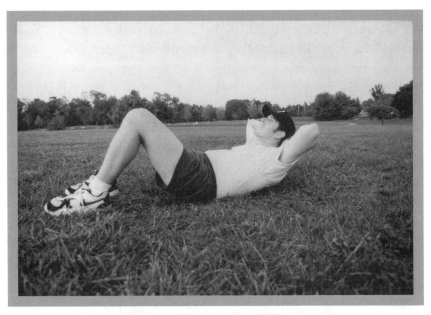

You can put your hands behind your head if you keep your chin up. (That's always good advice anyway.)

After a handful or a dozen or fifty, your neck may start to feel tight. Put your fingertips lightly behind your head and let your head rest in your hands. Don't pull from the arms. Imagine a crane anchored to your knees that has a hook into the middle of your chest. It's pulling your upper body toward your knees. Come up, take it down. Make sure you can fit a grapefruit underneath your chin.

Pull-ups

(When was the last time *you* climbed a tree?)

Pull-ups may be the toughest thing you do in Boot Camp. So, why bother? This is a major confidence-building exercise, as well as conditioning for your arms, shoulders, and back. Pulling is strong motion. Many people avoid activities that involve it, because they feel too weak to do it safely or effectively. If you do enough pull-ups to be able to handle tasks like these easily, your sense of accomplishment will soar:

Pull a full trash can down the driveway to the curb.

Pull yourself out of a chair.

Pull down the garage door.

Pull a big can of something off the shelf.

Pull down the hood of your car.

Pull down your attic ladder.

Remember: Pain is temporary, pride is forever.

Some of us remember what it was like to be a kid without a computer. We hung on to monkey bars and tree branches all day instead of joysticks; that's lots of pull-ups versus lots of repetitive strain injuries. As a result of this shift in juvenile pastimes, it's hard to find kids who can do pull-ups. Make them green with envy! Let them stare in awe as you pull yourself up to the top rung of a ladder!

We have two kinds of pull-ups in Boot Camp: A and B. For the memory-impaired, think, "Animal! I'm an animal!" and "Beast! I'm a beast!" You'll need a strong bar for each of these; the height depends on the level. Be prepared to improvise, and if you're lousy at

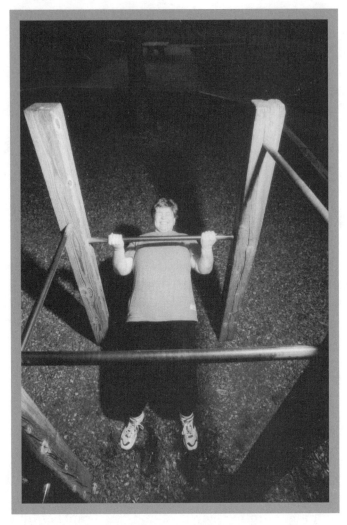

Let the assist give you a boost when the pull-up gets hard, but don't let your partner do all the work.

that, check out chapter 7. It has a handful of ideas on how to do pull-ups without playground equipment.

Pull-up A: When you walk up to the bar, it should hit you at the hips. That's because this pull-up does not require that you use your full body weight; you will rest some of your weight on your legs. Grasp the bar so your hands are just outside your hips, palms facing toward you. This puts your hands a little more than shoulder-width apart. Walk underneath the bar, so it's even with your chest.

With your knees bent slightly, pull your chest up to the bar, then lower it. If you need an assist, have your buddy squat behind you and help you reach the bar.

Pull-up B: This is done with your full body weight, but your buddy

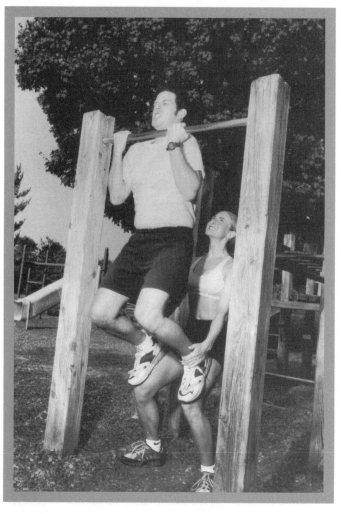

Bent legs make this exercise easier. Straighten the legs as you build up strength.

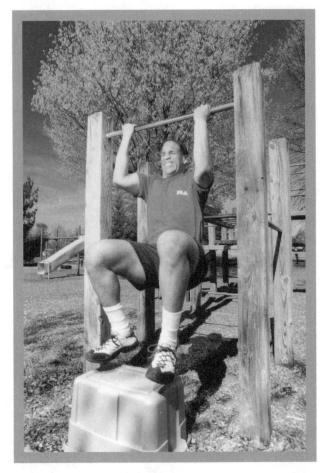

Slooowly let yourself down for the "negative." Exhale while you do it.

can assist you when you feel like there's lead in your butt. Grasp a bar that is low enough so you can reach it easily from the ground, but high enough so that you can dangle if your legs are slightly bent. Raise yourself so you can peek over the bar at the other kids in the playground, then lower yourself a little.

Don't let yourself drop all the way! I don't want you pulling your arms out of the socket. You'll look funny doing push-ups with your nose. Have your buddy stand behind you ready to give an assist at the waist.

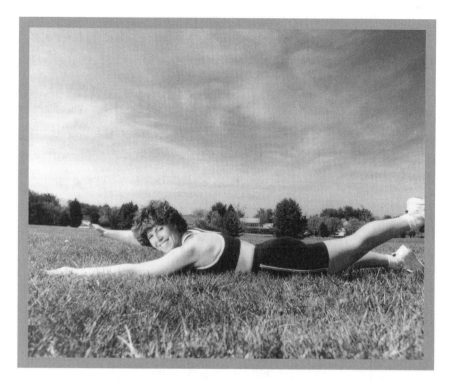

Look! In the field! It's Superman (or Superwoman)!

Here's a plan for working toward Pull-up B. If you can't find a buddy who wants to touch you, and you have trouble doing one pull-up on the high bar, put a chair or stool underneath the bar. Grab the bar with an underhand grip and put your chin(s) over it, as if you did the pull-up on your own power.

Bend your knees so your legs no longer support you and lower yourself slowwwwwly until your arms are extended. Don't drop! This type of exercise is called a "negative," but that doesn't mean it's worth less than nothing. Do these and eventually you WILL graduate to Pull-up B.

The Superman

(Strengthen your lower back and your gluteus-to-the-maximus.)

This is a really safe lower-back exercise that almost anyone can do. Take my word for it. It does not place a tremendous load on the

Dr. Bigbutt, M.D., was an Army major facing a periodic PT (physical training) test. She came to Boot Camp as a "refresher" in the basics. (That was her line of crap. She was fat and out of shape.) Unfortunately for her, she had a hard time showing up for class. Sergeant Lawrence called her a little after dawn and she had some lame excuse why she couldn't show up. Too bad for Dr. Bigbutt; it happened to be the same day that CBS-TV *This Morning* was taping workouts at Boot Camp.

Sergeant Lawrence took the camera crew and class to her house. The crew set up in her front yard at 0600 and lit it up like a shopping mall at Christmas. Class assembled and he barked, "One, two, argh, argh" as the Boots did push-ups outside her home.

Boom! Boom! Boom! He slammed his fist against her door. Dr. Bigbutt answered the door and stood there facing the camera—in her pajamas, nasty hair, but totally unshaken. Sergeant Lawrence was intense: "You have two minutes to get out here!"

She turned and left to follow orders, but never closed her door. So Sergeant Lawrence just followed her inside the house, and as she headed upstairs to dress, he took the camera crew into the kitchen. He opened the cupboard and found three cans of Pringle's potato chips, a big bag of cookies, some beer, and other goodies. He spread them all on the lawn for the world to see.

Dr. Bigbutt did a few penance push-ups that day. She also found no good reason to skip class again.

lower back, just enough to provide an effective workout. In fact, it is the only lower-back exercise that I personally do. And you all know why a strong back is important, don't you, gentle readers? Without it, you slouch over like a spineless wreck and can't even pick up the Sunday paper without taking eight hundred milligrams of ibuprofen. ("Ooohbooy, Marge, I really did it dis time. My back is killin' me!")

Eighty percent of my clients say they have bad backs: "My back is out, Sarge!" "Where did it go?" I ask. "Did it get pissed off at you and move out of the house? What do you mean, 'it's out?'" With most of them, it hurts sometime. It's generally not that bad, just weak or suffering from a slight muscle strain. Strengthen abs and erectors and keep them flexible—that's the cure.

Jane Brody, who writes about health issues for *The New York Times*, tells a classic story about her own lower-back pain.[3] Twenty years ago, she bent over to pick up a suitcase and couldn't stand up again. After a fruitless visit to the hospital, her doctor sentenced her to bed rest. Weeks went by and she asked, "Shouldn't I be exercising?" His answer, according to her, was, "You're not ready for that yet." Six weeks after her back "went out," she was told to begin exercising! The point she made in her column—loud and clear—is that "prolonged rest is just about the worst thing for both acute and chronic back problems." What you need is exercise. In fact, what you need is the superman.

Lay your body down with your face in the dirt. Extend your arms above your head. Raise your right arm and left leg six inches. Lift at the shoulder and at the hip. Lay them down slowly. Switch.

How many times do I have to tell you? Breathe while you do these exercises, so you look like you enjoy them. Or else!

Now it's time for you to do some more mental conditioning. Here is your homework.

ASSIGNMENT ONE

Go to a shopping mall and sit down for half an hour. Watch people shuffle from store to store. How many of them look tired? Log the number. Is shopping really all that tough that it wears out so many people? Look at the people struggling with their bags. Look at the different body postures from poor strength and flexibility.

---

[3] "Exercise prevents, helps heal back injuries," Jane Brody, October 1997.

People are bent over at hips and have tight lower backs—problems easily corrected with basic exercises. How many of them look out of shape? Log it. And whatever you do, don't say, "That one's fatter than me and so is that one over there."

You can do a similar exercise at an airport. The next time you're waiting for a flight, log the number of people who wheel a tiny bag instead of carrying it.

> As I pulled into the parking lot of the gym one day (Sarge also lifts weights), I noticed that a lady I'd seen before was parking in a handicapped spot. After scanning the car for the proper plates, stickers, or rearview mirror tag and seeing nothing, I asked her why she parked there. "I didn't want to walk too far." Then, I kid you not, young soldier, she went into the gym and immediately got on the treadmill. She later came to our offices to inquire about joining our Boot Camp program in Washington, D.C. I recognized her and she recognized me. We never heard from her again.

ASSIGNMENT TWO

While you're in Boot Camp (unless you get into a habit), I want you to:

- Carry your grocery bags whenever possible instead of driving the cart to your car.
- Park at the far end of the mall or a couple blocks from the restaurant when it's safe to do that.
- Mow your grass, scrub your floors, or do some other challenging chore around the house that you usually find someone else to do.
- Take the stairs in your building; if you're on a high floor, take half.
- Walk your dog. Get a dog if you don't have one.
- Wash and wax your own car.

- Walk to the store instead of driving.
- Go for a walk during your staff meeting; that is, make it a walking meeting, not a meeting you walk out of.

Now that you know how to do all the exercises—you can jog, you can stretch, you can activate those lazy muscles of yours in resistance training—you are nearly ready for Boot Camp. Twitching with excitement? You should be!

CHAPTER SEVEN
DO IT
ANYWHERE

Now that you know what to do, I'll tell you where to do it. As a taxpayer, you own a piece of the playground down the street, so consider your taxes health club dues. Same thing with the rent or mortgage on your home. If you already belong to a gym like the YMCA, fine. I can tell you how to use those facilities for your workout, too.

The bottom line is: It should cost you *nothing* extra to go through Boot Camp. You will use your own body weight for resistance—that means you develop muscle strength and endurance without hefting iron—and you will do this using ordinary benches, rods or bars, chairs, counter tops, floors, and stairs as "props." Give your bright pink tights to the meatheads in the gym (you better believe I don't want to see them) or to the Salvation Army and get down to basics! No music, no dancing, no mirrors, no machines, no spandex, no juice bars, no crybabies, no refunds!

AT THE PLAYGROUND

If you live in the suburbs or in a city that cares about its public lands, you will have a local playground where there is plenty of grass, gravel, mud, and dog crap. You will see monkey bars and jungle gyms. You will find stone benches, wooden benches, and wrought iron benches. And, unless you are in a densely populated urban environment, you will probably have access to a couple acres you can jog around safely.

I've built thousands of strong bodies using park land and playground equipment; that's primarily how my fitness program operates. When my instructors and I take recruits through Boot Camp, here is how we do it:

Standard or Modified Push-ups, Crunches, and Supermen

Any flat surface will do. It can be asphalt, loose stones, mud, or cool moss.

LISTEN UP!

The more unfit you are, the less weight you can push. That is why you may have to begin by doing push-ups against a wall. Imagine being arrested: That's the starting position. When you are ready, use a bench or other low object to put an angle into your push-up. Eventually, you WILL be strong enough to support your entire body weight and do push-ups on the deck (that's floor, civvies.)

Pam and her husband Richard, a large man known as Big Dick, reported to Boot Camp one fine cold March morning. She couldn't do one push-up, not even on her knees. I escorted her over to her new best friend—a back wall for tennis players—and had her do push-ups against the wall while her classmates got their noses dipped in the early morning frost. A year later, Pam was SuperPam (not to be confused with that oleo in a spray can), and Dick is now just Dick, running 10K road races. They're both loving life and she's wearing dresses in sizes she hadn't worn since he had hair.

Dips

Find yourself a park bench, a picnic table, or a high curb. Don't use your car bumper; your hands will slip off and your butt will end up on the street.

Pull-ups

Use a monkey bar like the ones you used to walk stiff-armed across when you were young and fit. Many playgrounds also have bars like the ones pictured in chapter 6. Use whichever level allows you to do the pull-up without having heart failure.

No matter where you're working out, you can always do a "negative" pull-up. Step up on a bench or stool under the bar so that your chin is over it, or get a boost up to the bar from your partner. The "negative" is lowering yourself down slowly. You can also do this kind of slow contraction if you are using a hip-high bar; either will help you build up to a regular pull-up. Take advantage of the negative and watch yourself get strong quickly.

Cardiorespiratory Workouts

Find a flat course where you can run or walk a mile or bike five miles.

At Boot Camp, my recruits know I get to class half an hour early whenever snow covers the ground. Everyone shows up those days because they know I'm such a hard-ass, that I'm out there digging out a track four feet wide by twenty yards long so they can exercise. If I could, I'd do that for you! The least you can do is dress appropriately and come outside, knowing that just getting your feet out the door puts you closer to fitness. Once you're out there, you'll feel like exercising.

Okay, so you live in Minnesota and sometimes it's pretty cold. I don't want anything to freeze and fall off. Here is what you can do.

AT HOME

If you can't find a floor space anywhere in your world that's big enough for your broad butt to stretch out, your world is too crowded. Throw out your La-Z-Boy—but please leave the plastic seat cover on—and make some room. And I don't want you working out in the middle of your kids' junk. Don't you dare send me whiny E-mail that you busted your hand on a Power Ranger.

Once you've made room to do your basic floor exercises like crunches and supermen away from the TV, here is how you approach the rest of the Boot Camp workout at home:

"Transition" Push-ups

(Those you do after graduating from push-ups against the wall, but before you're ready to do them on the floor.)

Locate a sturdy living room chair or couch, a nonrolling ottoman, or carpeted stairs.

- Lay a thick broomstick across the arms of a living room chair and push off of it. Make sure the stick is secure so you don't fall on your face.
- Do push-ups on your carpeted stairs. And listen, muffin-ass, I want your head pointed toward the top of the stairs, not the bottom. Start by doing your push-ups on a stair that's waist level. Place your feet flat on the ground. Put your hands shoulder-width apart on the stair that is waist high. Now, with your hands placed firmly on it, step back so your body is at a perfect forty-five-degree angle and push off. As you get stronger, work your way down the stairs until you get to the bottom step. If you're really weak and the stairway is narrow with handrails on both sides, you can do push-ups off the rails. Your hands should be directly under your shoulders, though, or you will hurt your shoulders and wind up unable to move your arms enough to wash your pits or blow-dry your hair.
- Use an ottoman (without casters) or push off the back of a couch that is set firmly against the wall.

Dips Inside the House

You're looking for a knee-high surface like a big chair or sofa that isn't going to move and is wide enough for you to put your hands shoulder-width apart. No dining room chairs—most are not wide or stable enough.

To use your sofa, take the cushions off and use the firm edge where your legs would normally be resting. Keep your shoes on your feet. If you're in stocking feet, you'll just slide around, not to mention stink up the whole house.

Dips Outside the House

Use your stoop steps or deck steps.

Pull-ups

Go to a sporting goods store and spend $19.99 on a solid chin-up bar you can put in a doorway.

Hook the chin-up bar low—hip height—as you start out. Remember the bent-knee rule: The tougher the pull-up gets, the more you bend the knees to keep going. Be sure to take the bar down when you're done so your kid doesn't do an end-over as she runs into the room. Wham! Slam! Instant gymnast!

Don't be cheap and try to use the door frame. First, your fingertips will scream bloody murder. Second, you lard asses could rip out the door frame. If you really can't afford the bar, look around outside your house for a well-secured bar or pipe that you can use for pull-ups.

Cardiorespiratory Workouts

If you want to stay inside, you'll need stairs or that treadmill or exercise bike you've been ignoring in your basement for six years. Outside, hit the sidewalk.

For your cardio workouts, don't be a dough boy (or girl). Get your lazy, musty-air breathin', junk-food eatin', couch-potato body out the door and walk, jog, or bike. Only under the most misery-making conditions should you consider staying in your comfy, cozy home.

When you do stay inside, here's the plan: Slowly climb the stairs in your house or in the stairwell of your apartment building. After you go up and down the stairs—holding the handrail, I might add—walk around your house or down the hall in your building, then hit the stairs again. Run in the house, sharp stick in the eye! (As a kid, my mother would always yell, "No running in the house, because if you do, you'll get a sharp stick in your eye!" Thanks, Mom, and thanks to all my buddies' moms, who must have picked up all the sharp sticks and hid them as we ran around the house. Not once did any of us get a sharp, or even a dull, stick in the eye.)

If you are doing a warm-up, keep moving slooooowly on those stairs for at least five minutes. On days when your focus is primarily the cardio workout, do this stairs-lap routine for fifteen to twenty minutes. At any time, if you feel dizzy or light-headed, sit down. Yup, sit right down on the stairs and continue to hold the handrail while you do, so you don't roll to the bottom of the stairwell and knock out a tooth. When you don't feel dizzy anymore, get off the stairs and stay off them. If you're in an apartment building, take the elevator back to wherever you belong.

After a couple days of walking up and down stairs, you will be so glad to jog, you will kiss the soles of your running shoes and yell, "Hallelujah, Sarge, gimme the great outdoors! I love snow! I love earthquakes! El Niño can kiss my grits!"

Did you think I forgot one really fun aerobic exercise—watching soap operas while running in place? Forget it, recruit. Don't run in place for more than the length of a commercial. It forces you to push off your toes, so it doesn't involve a natural running movement. I do not want you to get in the habit of running on your toes. Only cartoon characters and sissy aerobics instructors do that.

Don't run around your yard unless it's enormous. You'll look like a zoo animal. It might even make you so nuts you start yelling, "Let me out! Let me out!" Don't give the folks next door the idea that you should be locked up. The next thing you know, they'll start tossing peanuts over your fence and you'll have to put up a sign, NO FEEDING THE NEIGHBORS. (Of course, if they're willing to pay admission . . .)

IN THE GYM

If Boot Camp at home doesn't work because of noise or toys everywhere, maybe the only decent place you can exercise indoors is the local YMCA. No problem, recruit! You can go to a gym and find everything you need to do your complete Boot Camp workout. Just *stick with the program*, and don't walk into the barbells or the walking dumbbells. You know who I mean—those guys with the baggy leopard-skin pajamas and sweatshirts with no collars. When you have no neck, who needs a collar? And whoever told them they look good, anyway? ("Hey, Mom, wanna check out my new workout suit?" "Rocco, you look like you just stepped off the boat! Now get your tobacco-chewing, bad-haircut, worthless body up those stairs and put on the yellow tiger stripes!")

Rule number one for doing your Boot Camp workout in the gym is ignore what other people are doing. Go straight to the bench, mat, or treadmill that you need to do the job and do not let other people distract you.

Rule number two is try not to do all your workouts in the gym. Get some fresh air!

Standard or Modified Push-ups

Do them on the aerobics floor.

"Transition" Push-ups

Use a weight bench that is securely anchored.

Make sure you're doing your push-ups far away from those steroid monsters who fling dumbbells. If you hear a grunt, move.

Dips

Use a well-anchored weight bench.

Most gyms have dip bars, but I don't recommend you use them in Boot Camp. If you could safely do dips with your full body weight, you probably wouldn't be here.

Crunches and Supermen

Do them on the aerobics floor or a foam pad that the spandex crowd uses for stretching. (You can use it for stretching, too.)

Pull-ups

Look for the same kinds of bars as you would in a playground. If the only bar you find is high, use a solid bench or footstool underneath it to rest your feet on when you're done.

Many gyms also have a Gravitron machine that counterbalances your weight, so you can do pull-ups (and dips) with less than your body weight. If you use a machine like this, ask a certified trainer in the gym to show you how it works. Some of these machines are simple: Put the pin below the amount of weight you want to counterbalance yours. The more plates you use, the easier the exercise. Others do the counterbalancing with air pressure, and you need a degree in computer science to figure them out.

Cardiorespiratory Workouts

Take a jog on a treadmill.

A treadmill distributes the load—your load—more evenly than stair climbers and some other fancy machines, so I prefer it to other aerobic devices. Of course, if you really enjoy riding that stationary bike into the sunset, sit your big butt down and go for it. But while you're there in the cardio room of the gym, take a good whiff of the perfume, garlic breath, and farts all around you. You'll be so happy to breathe fresh air after that, I guarantee you will never again use weather as an excuse not to jog outside.

PLACES AND THINGS TO AVOID

Here are a few other don't-do-this-or-you'll-regret-it tips that apply throughout Boot Camp:

- Don't do pull-ups off your deck. The wood can be weakened by weather. It will split and you'll fall on the ground and break your neck; then you'll go to the doctor, who'll collaborate with your lawyer, and you'll present me with a lawsuit. Then what, you worthless bag of atrophy? My publisher will hate me so I won't be able to write any more books. I'll have to sell my house; I won't be able to feed my wife or child or my dog Snyper; I'll have to shut down my business; and I'll probably have to jump off a bridge because I won't be able to live my dream anymore. Worst of all, the rest of the world will not receive the love and attention that you have received from me. All because you didn't listen. So listen to me!
- Don't do push-ups facing downhill. You could strain your shoulders. See above result.
- Don't do dips on parallel bars that are wider than 2½ feet or you'll strain your shoulder. See above result.
- Don't do the superman on a hill. You could roll down it, smashing dog crap and hurting your shoulders. See above result.
- Don't do dips off lawn furniture. Don't do dips on anything your two-year-old can throw around. See above result.
- Don't run on hills during these first three weeks of Boot Camp. You're not ready yet; it could cause shin splints. See above result.

- Don't do crunches on the downhill. It's too easy. Don't do them uphill, either, at least until you've graduated.
- And men, do the superman on a soft surface. If you can't find a carpeted or grassy area, put a donut between your legs so you don't hurt yourself. Don't even think about doing this exercise on concrete or, worse yet, gravel.

No matter where you go or how you improvise, apply safety and common sense—got it?

CHAPTER EIGHT

REVEILLE!

Get your loaf out of bed! This is the time to dust off your Polaroid and take "before" pictures of that gelatinous blob you call a body.

How did you sleep last night? A little restless? Good. It means you're excited. You should be; you are about to change your life forever.

Here you are on the first day wearing a brand new pair of sneakers. You've got your tall socks on, your shorts are pulled up to your chest, and your shirt's tucked in. You're so wired. If I yell "pushups," you'll push so high it'll look like you're humping the air. If I

Homer had never exercised; he had a dozen ways to get out of Phys Ed in school. On the first day of Boot Camp, he came dragging his gut and looking for a place to sit down. His hope was that someone would get him moving so he could play with his three young sons. When I began administering the fitness test, I ordered all the new recruits to get ready to do push-ups continuously for two minutes and count them. "Down!" I barked. "Readyyyy, set—" Suddenly, he looked up at me with this big grin taking up most of his big, bald head and asked, "How many do you want me to do, Sarge?" I snarled, "What do you mean, 'How many?' How many can you do?" "Two," he said, still grinning. It occurred to me this guy had no clue what he was getting himself into. "Then do ten more!" I snapped. Guess what? He did fifteen.

tell you to jog, you'll sprint. Hold on to that, recruit! You are about to be reborn; you are about to rediscover the best part of your childhood. The first day of Boot Camp is your first step toward more fun than you've had in years!

Before we begin, be prepared in these five ways:

- Look at your watch. What time is it? This is the time you will work out every day. You need consistency so exercise becomes a habit, and I will be there to enforce it: If you are ever late, you automatically owe me an extra twenty push-ups—no excuses! I prefer a dawn workout and you will, too, recruit. You want me in your face every morning; that's why you're in Boot Camp.

- Treat yourself to a "Sarge's Private Moment" before the workout. Every day before I train, I grab the most recent issue of *Time* magazine and go to the most important room in my house. I stay there until I'm done and you will, too. If you don't, you will have to use the bushes during your jog.

- Be prepared with a full water bottle and a towel. Babies can use a blanket.

- Wear running shoes every day. I don't mean cross-trainers or tennis shoes or penny loafers. As I have explained before, running shoes have a special construction that you need for this program. Expect your shoes to get wet some days. Deal with it.

> Kevin, a 350-pound dude, showed up for Boot Camp wearing blue $7.95 sneakers he had bought at the grocery store. You know the kind—a Velcro strap over some cheap plastic. I didn't have to make fun of him because everyone else did, but I did anyway. The next day, he had decent shoes.

- Dress appropriately. First of all, that means wear clothing you can get dirty. Second, you will need a couple layers of clothing when it's cold, but these layers must wick moisture away from your body, not hold it next to you. Synthetics work best; I recommend talking with an intelligent person at the local sports-clothing store to get advice on what is best for your climate.

Avoid cotton in wet and cold weather, because it will make you miserable. Third, what do you do when it's raining? Wear a hat, Einstein. If you insist on doing the workout inside your house, wear the hat anyway in honor of those brave, committed recruits who are outside. You never know when you'll get the urge to join the rest of us. Fourth, if you sweat heavily, you will be more comfortable in socks made of a polyester-nylon blend rather than cotton. Wear them up to your knees so I can identify you as I drive through your neighborhood. The synthetic material may have some highfalutin brand name like Fungus-Be-Gone, but whatever its called, it will keep your stinky feet from getting any more disgusting. And don't be like Fred, the guy who works in our office: Change your socks every day.

> A thirty-five-year-old lawyer, who had acquired a hefty circle of flab since law school, wrote in his log about the first week of Boot Camp: "We ran in the cold. We ran in the dark. We ran in the freezing rain. We did push-ups and stomach crunches in the mud. I thought it was a great experience."

Finally, a reminder: Get yourself a buddy for Boot Camp. You *want* someone who will call you when you feel lazy and bark, "Get your fat can out of the rack. It's raining! Hoooraahhh!"

> Don wanted somebody to run with; it was the only part of Boot Camp he really had a hard time motivating himself to do. On Day Five, he paired up with a woman who was determined to lose weight, just like he was. Unfortunately, she hated running more than he did. She was ready to give up almost immediately. Don kept psyching her up for the next step, then the next tenth of a mile, until they finished the run. They laughed and decided they would be a good team for the next two weeks. Later, Don thought to himself, "What am I—a fruitcake? I thought I hated running."

> The moral of this story is: Be a fruitcake. Find someone to help you through this and buy the book for him or her. You'll have more fun and help make this book a best-seller.

There are also two things you will never do in Boot Camp. I have my reasons. I might even tell you what they are.

- You will never wear things that can distract or get in your way during exercise. One example is headphones. You need to focus on your breathing and your body alignment, not whatever you call music. It could also reduce your environmental awareness so you step off a curb and into a speeding tricycle. Another example is jewelry. Wear a watch and any other essential gear like a drug-reaction bracelet or wedding ring, but leave the fancy junk in your drawer at home.

- You will not stop to take your pulse. During Boot Camp, the measure of how you pace yourself will be "perceived exertion," and you can refer to the following chart called the Ratings of Perceived Exertion, or Borg chart.[1] Recommended by the American College of Sports Medicine, this method of determining how hard you can push relies on common sense, not numbers. Can you handle that?

  Perceived exertion is a personal way of measuring the difficulty of an exercise. If it is very hard to do a single push-up, you might rate it as a 17 on this scale. If you have no trouble climbing ten stairs but are breathing harder and feel it offered some challenge, you might rate it an 11. I want you a little higher than middle range for these exercises; that is, stay within 12 to 16 in the level of difficulty. The only time you are allowed to exceed the middle range is on test day, but I never want you pushing so hard you pass out on me!

---

[1] The Ratings of Perceived Exertion were developed by G. V. Borg (1982). There is also a 10-point scale, as well as the original 6–20-point scale. On the 10-point version, 0 represents "nothing at all," 1 is "very weak," 2 is "weak," 3 is "moderate," then the intensities increase incrementally to 10, which is "very, very strong."

RATINGS OF PERCEIVED EXERTION

1–4 You are asleep, at your desk at work, or watching *Wheel of Fortune.*

5 You're wiggling your toes with your loafing, fat ass sitting in a chair.

6 What are you doing? Walking from the deli counter to your table?

7 Very, very light

8 You're channel surfing manually and have to stretch to reach the TV controls.

9 Very Light

10 You're starting to feel a little sweaty, but you don't stink yet.

11 Fairly light

12 Now you're working! You're in Boot Camp territory!

13 Somewhat hard

14 Starting to stink . . .

15 Hard

16 Really stinkin'. You'll feel this tomorrow and be glad, recruit!

17 Very hard

18 Easy, soldier! Don't kill yourself in MY program.

By the way, Borg's real descriptions are **bolded** on this chart, whereas The Sarge's editorial comments are not.

Be prepared Monday through Friday in all the above ways. Monday, Wednesday, and Friday workouts involve the same sequence of exercises; they are focused on your muscular strength, muscular endurance, and flexibility. Tuesday and Thursday are your aerobic training days with a stretching session at the beginning.

You will get Saturdays and Sundays off, but if you want a head start on your buddies, walk briskly for thirty minutes at least one of those days.

We're ready to begin, so make sure your shoes are tied and stop picking your nose. You will call me Sarge from now on, whether you know me socially or not. If I tell a joke, you will laugh. If you tell a joke, I may or may not laugh, depending on my mood. If your joke stinks, you will drop and give me twenty. (P.S. I like short jokes so I don't have to pay attention very long.)

This is it, recruit!

DAY ONE

45-minute workout:

10-minute warm-up, 2-minute cooldown, 8 minutes of stretches, 15 minutes for exercises with stretching in between exercises, 8-minute jog, and 2-minute cooldown

Warm-Up

At a slow pace, jog half a mile. Alternatively, you can walk it briskly. This will take about ten to twelve minutes. Stay alert, breathe consistently, and remain comfortable.

Singing to yourself can help you set a pace anytime you jog or power walk. I do it all the time. I sing military chants as I run down the road with a big smile on my face. People think I'm a nut. Are you surprised? Try it, but if your brain runs out of songs, repeat after me:

LISTEN UP!

With the cadence, take two half breaths so you inhale during the words; exhale in two half breaths after the phrase. The breathing should correspond to your foot striking the ground. Repeat with each phrase.

I'm the Sarge (step, step)

Takin' charge (step, step)

You're with me (step, step)

Feelin' free (step, step)

Breathin' light (step, step)

Gettin' tight (step, step)

Hatin' lard (step, step)

Runnin' hard (step, step)

P T (step, step)

With me (step, step)

Awwl day (step, step)

Can't wait (step, step)

Awwl night (step, step)

Awwl right (step, step)

Feels good (step, step)

Looks good (step, step)

Look at me (step, step)

Look at you (step, step)

Runnin' hard (step, step)

With the Sarge (step, step)

He's the man (step, step)

With the plan (step, step)

Eating fruit (step, step)

What a brute (step, step)

I said up in the morning with the rising sun

Runnin' and gunnin' and havin' fun.

Butt-sniffin' dog don't get in my way

I'm runnin' hard, no time to play.

The Sarge is mean and the Sarge is good

whippin' ass in our neighborhood.

Hey, old lady, lookin' at me

Stop your starin', start runnin' with me.

Momma, momma, can't you see

What PT has done for me?

Got up early and took a pee

Now I'm gonna be all I used to be.

You can make things up as you go along, but no swearing.

Cooldown

Walk around for a couple minutes and get your breathing back to normal. Drink some water.

Sit Down

Put your blanket between you and the ground. Sit on it.

Stretch

I said, "Sit down!" This week as you're getting used to the routine, review the description of each stretch before you try it. It is very important that you understand what your body is supposed to do before you do it. Never—I'm serious now—*never* force your body into a stretch. For example, if merely sitting in the correct position for a hamstring stretch is the maximum you can do, then that's what you do today.

Remember to breathe while you do these stretches. If you don't breathe, you will burst a blood vessel. You think I'm kidding? Have you ever held your breath while trying to push a heavy piece of furniture or lift a large object (or human)? Bearing down without breathing is called a Valsalva maneuver, and it can send your blood pressure through the roof. It can also cause hemorrhoids. (By the way, a Valsalva maneuver isn't always deadly. If you're trying to adjust to an altitude change or you're scuba diving, you can use it to adjust middle ear pressure.)

I said, "Breathe!"

Start off by giving your lower back a treat.

Lower-Back Stretch
1 x 30 seconds

REVIEW: LOWER-BACK STRETCH

Legs crossed "Indian style." Arch your back, lean forward, and drop your head.

Time to stretch the back of your thighs.

Seated Hamstring Stretch
2 x 30 seconds (that's twice for 30 seconds, private)

REVIEW: HAMSTRING STRETCH

Legs in front with toes together in the air. Back straight; reach toward toes.

Make sure you hold the stretch without bouncing. Hoorah, let's do it: thirty, twenty-nine, twenty-eight, a bunch of other numbers, five, four, three, two, one. Relax. Repeat this.

If you're too fat in the legs to put them together, just open them up a little to do the exercise. Let your gut fall down between them. We'll deal with that later.

Work those flabby inner thighs—now!

Straddle Stretch
1 x 30 seconds

REVIEW: STRADDLE STRETCH

Legs spread, toes pointed up. Reach forward as far as you can in between your legs.

Remember, if your legs are already apart during the hamstring stretch, move them even further out. And hold that stretch when

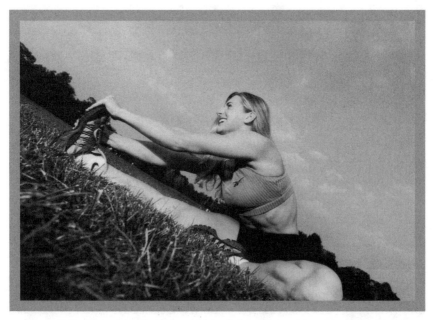

Easy does it—no bouncing. Ahhh, it feels great to clean your toes.

you reach forward: thirty, twenty-nine, whatever, nine, eight, seven, six, five, four, three, two, one, one. Did I put an extra one in there? You can handle it.

I'm going to add a little variation now. Stretch to the left as if you are trying to reach your left toe. Then stretch to the right.

Left Straddle Stretch
1 x 30 seconds

Right Straddle Stretch
1x 30 seconds

Go back to the hamstring stretch and focus on one leg at a time, gently reaching for that big toe or knee or whatever you can find.

Right Hamstrings stretch
1 x 30 seconds

Left Hamstrings Stretch
1 x 30 seconds

Go back to working on the lower back and get your gluteus maximus in the action.

Sergeant's Salute (Gluteal/Lower-Back Stretch)
1 x 30 seconds

REVIEW: THE SERGEANT'S SALUTE

On your back, legs slightly apart. Pull knees into the chest; butt in the air.

Just like the other ones, hold this stretch. C'mon, reeeecruit, I want to see the bottom of your big butt pointing at me!

Now repeat the first stretch you did.

Lower-Back Stretch
1 x 30 seconds

That slab of meat in the front of your legs needs help, too.

Right Quadriceps Stretch
1 x 30 seconds

Left Quadriceps Stretch
1 x 30 seconds

REVIEW: QUAD STRETCH

Stand up. Press forward with the pelvis, then pull one leg back by grabbing the ankle.

If you're really good, you can do a jump change to grab the other leg. As you let one leg down, hop as you bend the other one up. If you're coordinated, you'll save time. If not, your face will end up in the dirt.

Time to loosen up your chest and shoulders—work those pectoral muscles and anterior deltoids.

POW Stretch (Upper Body)
1 x 30 seconds

REVIEW: POW STRETCH

Stand. Put fingertips together behind your head, elbows out. Put chin to chest.

Hold your position and squeeeeeze those shoulder blades together.

You'll need your arms for push-ups, recruit, so let's wake them up.

Arm Circles and Finger Crunches
1 x 10 seconds in each direction

> **REVIEW: ARM CIRCLES AND FINGER CRUNCHES**
>
> Slightly bend arms and rotate them in ever-widening circles. Wiggle fingers; squeeze.

While you roll your arms in a count of ten for both directions, keep your digits moving at the same time. It doesn't take too much coordination to do these two things at once.

You've made it all the way to the head. Good work. Let's get some flexibility in your shoulder girdle, upper back, and neck.

Shrugs
2 x 10 seconds

> **REVIEW: SHRUGS**
>
> Hands at rest on the quadriceps. Elevate shoulders toward ears and drop them slowly.

Ten, nine, eight, seven, you can count the rest.

Welcome to the last stretch. By now, your nickname is "rubber band."

Neck Turns
1 x 10 seconds in each direction

> **REVIEW: NECK STRETCH**
>
> Eyes right, hold. Eyes left, hold. Drop your chin on your chest.

Remember to hold for ten seconds each time you turn. And when I say "eyes right," soldier, that doesn't mean just your eyes. Do something with your head, too, otherwise this isn't a neck stretch. When you drop your chin, say a prayer, because your next move is a push-up!

Push-ups

The arms and chest will now report to Boot Camp.

First try the exercise on your toes—the standard push-up—as described in chapter 6. Only if you honestly rank this in the "very hard" range on the Perceived Exertion scale should you begin at the knee position (modified push-up), on a bench or stair (transition push-up), or against a wall. Be sure to cross the ankles and bring the heels into the butt for the modified push-up. This keeps your body weight off your kneecaps and shifts it to your thighs.

To maintain good body position in this exercise, pretend a two-by-four is tied to you from your head down to your toes. That means your body is straight and stiff as you do the push-up. What are the three points on your body that come toward the ground simultaneously, recruit? Nose, nipples, and navel. Good! There's hope for you.

When you start shaking like a leaf as you do the push-up, drop down to the knee position. At this point, you've reached the "very hard" level, and I want you to stay in the middle range. Cross your ankles when you move into the knee position. Bring your nose, navel, and nipples toward the ground again. Notice I said "toward." I want you close to the ground, not eating it.

This week, you'll do twenty-five push-ups. Do a combination of standard, modified, and any other kind until you get there. One way or another, get to the *target twenty-five*. Even if you don't make the number, do the best you can. You never know, I might be watching.

After-Push-up Stretch

Stand up. Put your hands behind your head and stretch your pectoral and shoulder muscles again in a count of ten.

POW Stretch
1 x 30 seconds

You WILL stretch after each strength-building exercise, so pay attention.

Jog or Brisk Walk

We're going to take a jog or brisk walk for ten minutes. If you begin with a jog but start breathing heavily, take it down to a walk. I don't want you racing ahead of me. You'll impress me a whole lot more with easy breathing than you will with sweat pouring off your forehead.

Cool Down

Walk around and get your breathing back to normal. Drink some water.

Dips

It's time to work on your bingo arms. That flabby part that hangs down when you raise your arm is part fat, part floppy triceps muscle. "It" is really "they" because the triceps has three components, and you're going to work every one of them.

REVIEW: DIPS

Hands over the edge of the bench. Keep arms steady; lower yourself then come up.

One repetition is one dip. With each one, you should feel the exercise in the back of your arms. If you don't, you're doing it wrong. Do one set to failure. For you civvies new to fitness, that means "do as many as you can."

If this is too easy, place your legs out a little farther. If that's still easy, go up on your heels.

I often see people with their butts a mile away from the bench. Don't do that! Stay close. If you use a chair, do not put your hands on the side of the chair. If you slip, you could break your arms or rip your shoulder socket.

The shoulder is a very vulnerable, unstable joint. If you do an ex-

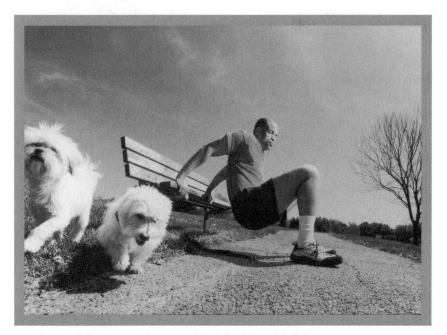

I scared the dogs when I yelled at Fred for his bad form. Now, keep your butt close to the bench or I'll scare you, too.

ercise like the bench dip improperly, you will fall down and go "boom." You'll end up in surgery. Six months later you might think about exercising again, but then you'll have forty extra pounds on you and be so disgusted and discouraged that you won't do it. You'll succumb to all the weebles in the world who find reasons not to sweat. Don't go there!

After-Dip Stretch

You worked your triceps twice now—once with push-ups and once with dips. Time to stretch this area. Take your right arm and place it in the air. Bend your arm behind your head so the fingertips are touching the back of your neck and your elbow is pointed in the air. Take the opposite hand and grab the elbow that's pointing upward; hold it as close to your head as possible. Don't forget to breathe; we don't want any hemorrhoids!

Hold for ten, nine, eight, seven, whatever. Now switch arms. Be sure you bring the elbow to the head, not the head to the elbow. This is when you really feel how high your shorts can go.

Left Triceps Stretch
1 x 10 seconds

Right Triceps Stretch
1 x 10 seconds

The only thing I don't like about this stretch is that it always hikes my shorts up and makes me look like Little Lord Fauntleroy, or for you TV watchers, Martin Short's dorky Ed Grimley character. I hate it when I look silly. Are you laughing at me just thinking

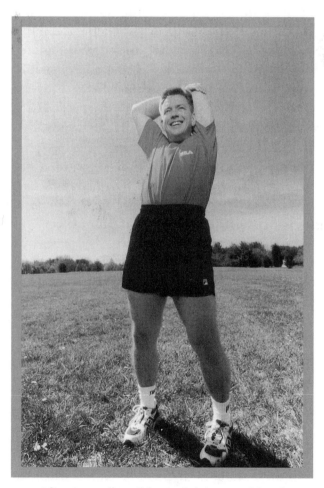

After your dips, this stretch is your friend.

about it? I always adjust my shorts before I do that stretch, otherwise people won't take me seriously when I yell, "Give me twenty!"

Crunches

> ### REVIEW: CRUNCHES
>
> Bent legs, feet shoulder-width apart. Lift upper back off ground, squeeze abs, lower.

Find a spot on the grass, preferably not where your dog has been. Lie down. It's time to work your abdominal muscles. This will not (hear me? *not*) get rid of fat around your middle. This will give the muscles in that area tone, strength, and shape, so when you stop eating junk and the blubber is gone, you just might have a six-pack. For those of you new to exercise, a six-pack is the gorgeous abdominal definition that shows up on shows like *Baywatch.*

There is no such thing as "lower abs" or "upper abs," so you don't need three different exercises to work your abdominals. Crunches work all areas of your abdominal muscles, which run from the area of your fifth rib (counting from the top) to your pelvis.

Don't get lazy: Contract your abdominals—squeeze your stomach muscles as if you're bearing down—when you lift your upper back off the ground. (No Valsalva maneuver, though!) Lower yourself back down to the ground slowly. That means you're in control, not out of control, soldier. Come up again and squeeze. How many is that? Two. Good!

Do it again, and when you do, I don't want to see you bringing your chin into your chest. Keep your face parallel to the ground. Try it again. That's three. Do a few more: four, five, six, seven, eight, nine, ten. Good! Use your fingertips to assist you only after your neck starts to feel tight.

For those who are completely new to crunches, once you do about fifteen, they will become painful. This is when the fun begins. Think about pizza. Have visions of doughnuts. This is when I want you to focus on all the fattening food you have eaten. While you're doing these crunches and you're in excruciating pain—and have thirty-five more to go, I want you to imagine eating greasy French fries. Every time you come up, think about stuffing your face with fried chicken and buttered bread. Open your mouth as you feel like screaming in pain and imagining putting a hunk of chocolate cake in there. Smell pizza as you breathe more heavily. Close your eyes and see the cheese dripping off the side. Do a close-up of the pizza in your mind so that you see every fat molecule. All of a sudden it changes into the biggest, fattest butt and thighs in the world, and it's right in front of your face about to sit on you!

We're done with crunches. Good work.

> On her first day in Boot Camp, Carol missed the instructions for the crunch, because she was distracted. Her spot was a patch of mud and wet grass, and she wasn't happy about that. By the time Sergeant Ahmad reached her, she had already done at least ten "crunches," several more than anyone else in the class.
>
> When she found out she had to move more than her head, though, she couldn't do them quite so fast anymore.
>
> Guess what she learned? Crunches are not neck-ups.

After-Crunch Stretches

Once again, we're going to stretch after working a major muscle group. While you're still on the ground, lengthen your body as if you're Superman. Drop your legs down and put your arms straight above you. Breathe in using your stomach muscles, then let it come out. This is called diaphragmatic breathing, for you geeks. Breathe in, really trying to expand your ribs, then breathe out. Do this about ten times, but don't do it so fast and so deep that you pass out. I don't want anyone discovering your limp body with a copy of this book next to you. If you're going to pass out, hide the book first.

Now that you're here we're going to stretch the lower back. Pull into a sergeant's salute. Pull your knees into your chest, put your butt in the air, and wave it like you just don't care. If you have a lot of bulk (i.e., stomach) in the front, pull your knees apart and make room for it.

Sergeant's Salute
1 x 30 seconds

Pull-ups: Modified and Standard

REVIEW: PULL-UPS

Pull-up A: Bar is hip height. With knees bent, pull chest to the bar; slowly lower it.

Pull-up B: High bar. Raise body weight so chin is above the bar; slowly lower it.

If you are carrying an extra forty or fifty pounds, a standard pull-up (pull-up B) might be too tough for you. Heck, it's probably tough if you're at a good weight and just aren't used to it. Pick the one you can do for at least fifteen repetitions. If you can do any standard pull-ups, do as many as you can, then go to the modified ones and continue. I'd rather see you on your back for the pull-up than on your back in a hospital bed after pulling your arm out of the socket. (I hate to buy flowers except for my wife, and you *know* I'm not bringing you candy; so don't end up in the hospital.) Just remember to do this move slowly. I like to use a four-count: Up is one thousand one, one thousand two, one thousand three, one thousand four, then down to the same count. You WILL get tired, and you WILL build strength quickly.

For pull-up A, pull your chest up to the bar, then lower it. Up, then lower. Do it again and again. If you need an assist, have your buddy squat behind you—that's squat, not bend—and help you reach the bar.

Was that too easy for you? Straighten out your legs, then do the exercise. Better yet, begin pull-up A with straight legs, then bend them as you get wimpy.

If you do pull-up B, there are two big things to remember if you want my respect:

1. Do not let yourself drop all the way.
2. If your buddy is male, do not let your feet flail when he assists you. Don't kick him in his thinking spot.

After-Pull-up Stretches

Arms up and slightly out to the sides. Now bend at the elbows and touch your head. Pretend you're grabbing a beach ball on the

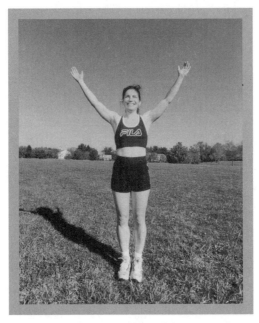

Raise your arms up to the sky like a big "Y."

side. Arms up with the fingertips touching. You fell for this, didn't you? You are just like the Wingnut, my coauthor! Were you asleep during the seventies? Truthfully, everyone falls for this one. I'm so clever.

This is the real stretch: Put your left arm in the air. Grab it at the wrist with your right hand. Lean to your right, stretching your latissimus dorsi, the muscle in the upper part of the back that flares out

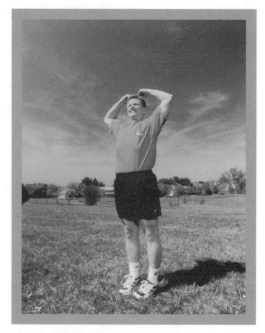

Fingertips on the head, a little like an "M."

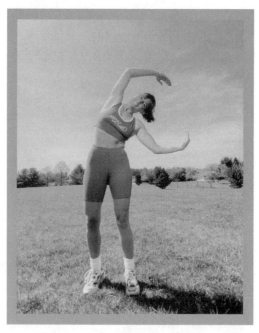

Bend to side and pretend to grab a beachball.
Your arms are like a big "C."

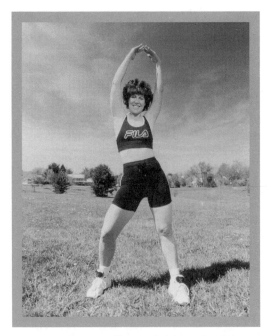

Haven't you figured this out YET?

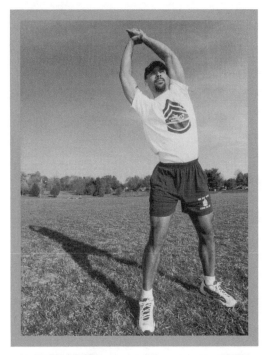

Stretch to the side, but don't bend yourself in half.

like a meaty wing on bodybuilders. Switch arms and stretch to the left, because the latissimus dorsi happens to be on both sides of your spine.

Right Lat Stretch
1 x 30 seconds

Left Lat Stretch
1 x 30 seconds

While you're still standing, put your fingertips together, and with your head down, stretch forward with your back rounded.

Upper-Back Stretch
1 x 30 seconds

The Superman

REVIEW: SUPERMAN

Lie face down, arms extended above head. Raise right arm, left leg, then switch sides.

You will aim for a total of twenty; that's a measly ten on each side. Do whatever you want with your head except twist it around.

After-Superman Stretches
Slide your butt down to your heels. Walk your fingertips so they pull your arms away from your body as much as possible. Relax. Have a seat and spread your legs.

Left Straddle Stretch
2 x 10 seconds

Right Straddle Stretch
2 x 10 seconds

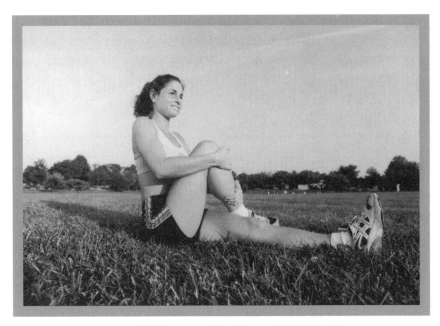

Do this in a way that's comfortable.
If your foot won't go up this far, don't force it.

Relax between stretches. If you can't reach your toes with your fin-gertips, touch something higher up on your leg.

Cross your right leg over your left, then take your right arm and wrap it around the knee. With your left hand, grab your sock and pull your leg tight into your body. Do this at a level that is comfort-able. Keep your back straight. Switch: Left leg over the right, left hand over the knee, grab your sock with your right hand, and pull the leg. This stretches your buttocks—the gluteus maximus, that bulky part of the butt, the big cheeseball—the thing that will give us great joy. Why?

Tight butts drive 'em nuts
Ain't no junk in that trunk!

Right Gluteal Stretch
1 x 30 seconds

Left Gluteal Stretch
1 x 30 seconds

Time to stretch the lower back again. Sit Indian style with legs crossed. This time, wrap your arms underneath your legs, grab your toes, and bring your head down, pulling your chest to your legs. Relax, then sit up.

Lower-Back Stretch
1 x 30 seconds

Grab your partner. Tell your partner to grab you. Put an arm around each other's shoulder. Grab the opposite leg. If your partner is grabbing a left leg, you're grabbing your right. Keep your knees next to each other and shift your pelvis forward. Pull the leg back. Both of you should be leaning forward a bit, looking like the FTD florist symbol. Turn around and face the other way and work the opposite leg.

Right Quadriceps Stretch
1 x 30 seconds

Left Quadriceps Stretch
1 x 30 seconds

If you don't have a partner, grab a pole, or a tree, or an innocent by-stander. Just say, "Hey! Come here! Hold me up so my face doesn't end up in dog turds!"

This class is ended. Go in peace. Your homework is to walk twenty minutes, then do the hamstrings stretch, the lower-back stretch, and the quadriceps stretch.

DAY TWO

45-minute workout: 5-minute warm-up, 2-minute cooldown, 8 minutes of stretches, 20-minute aerobic workout, 5-minute cooldown, 5 minutes of crunches and supermen

Welcome back, recruit! You're an animal! Yesterday was primarily a resistance workout for your upper body. Today, your main focus is your cardiorespiratory system, and if you jog or walk, you'll be using your legs a lot. If you can't jog or walk, put yourself on a bike or go swimming.

Warm-up

Take a walk. Jog when you feel like it. Do it for five minutes. You could also pull some weeds in your yard or pick up your (kid's) toys.

Stretch

After your warmup, go through the sequence of stretches:

Lower-back stretch	1 x 30 seconds
Seated hamstrings stretch	2 x 30 seconds
Straddle stretch	1 x 30 seconds
Left straddle stretch	1 x 30 seconds
Right straddle stretch	1 x 30 seconds
Right hamstrings stretch	1 x 30 seconds
Left hamstrings stretch	1 x 30 seconds
Sergeant's salute (gluteal stretch)	1 x 30 seconds
Lower-back stretch	1 x 30 seconds
Right quadriceps stretch	1 x 30 seconds
Left quadriceps stretch	1 x 30 seconds
POW stretch (upper body)	1 x 30 seconds
Arm circles and finger crunches	1 x 10 seconds each direction
Shrugs	2 x 10 seconds
Neck turns	1 x 10 seconds each direction

Jog or Walk

Hit the trail again. Make your walk brisk. Make your run light. Enjoy breathing. You are moving toward fitness and you're going to go in that direction for twenty to twenty-five minutes. I'm right there, making strange remarks as you and your friend jog through the park, so you better go the full time or you're busted!

On the third day of Boot Camp, a woman approached her sergeant on duty very shyly. She whispered, "I have not had a bowel movement in two days. Does Boot Camp make you constipated?" He was surprised. "No, ma'am. I find it accelerates nature." The next day she arrived at Boot Camp with a smile. She took him aside and said, "You were right! I had three last night!" "Okaaay," he muttered. "A little more information than I needed, but thanks for keeping me informed."

Cooldown

Walk around until you're breathing normally. Drink water. Don't skip this stuff, recruit. The purpose of a cooldown is to prevent dizziness, fainting, and other problems that can result from stopping vigorous exercise too abruptly. You've just moved quickly for twenty to twenty-five minutes, unless you cheated. You need about five minutes now to get your blood vessels and lungs calmed down. Do what I tell you!

Crunches

Every day is an abs day, right, recruit? Do one set of crunches, starting with your arms crossed in front of you, and aim for fifty. You may be so sore from yesterday that you don't even do as many today. Don't worry—it probably means you did them right!

The Superman

Aim for twenty. And remember, guys, don't do this one on concrete or you will be singing soprano. Women, this won't help you sing soprano.

DAY THREE

45-minute workout: 10-minute warm-up, 2-minute cooldown, 8 minutes of stretches, 15 minutes for exercises with stretching in between exercises, 8-minute jog, and 2-minute cooldown

Welcome back! You have nothing new to learn, just a few more of everything to do because you have more energy and strength! You are an ace recruit! Hoooraahhh!! Here's a recap, because as you've noticed, I like to make things convenient for you:

- Warm up: At a slow pace, jog or walk half a mile. Breathe in and out in a four-count.
- Cool down: Grab your water bottle and use it.
- Stretch: Check out the list for Day Two. That's what you need; that's what you do every day in Boot Camp.
- Push-ups: Give me twenty-five.
- After–push-up stretch: POW stretch (1 x 30 seconds).
- Jog for ten minutes; turn this into a walk if you have to gasp for air.
- Cool down again.
- Dips: Do as many as you can.
- After-dip stretch: Left and right triceps stretch (each one held ten seconds). Check your pants. This is the one that pulls up your drawers.
- Crunches: You're still aiming for fifty.
- After-crunch stretches: Breathe deeply while you're on your back, then do the sergeant's salute (1 x 30 seconds).
- Pull-ups: I said fifteen, recruit.
- After–pull-up stretches: Right and left lat stretches (30 seconds each) that move right into the upper-back stretch, with finger-tips together in front of you, and your head down (30 seconds).
- The superman: All I want is ten on each side.
- After-superman stretches: You're almost done now. Left and right straddle stretches, left and right gluteal stretches, the lower-back stretch, and left and right quadriceps stretch (each one held 30 seconds).
- Walk a little while to cool down and congratulate yourself.

DAY FOUR (SAME AS DAY TWO)

45-minute workout:	5-minute warm-up, 2-minute cooldown, 8 minutes of stretches, 20-minute aerobic workout, 5-minute cooldown, 5 minutes of crunches and supermen

DAY FIVE (SAME AS DAYS ONE AND THREE)

45-minute workout: 10-minute warm-up, 2-minute cooldown, 8 minutes of stretches, 15 minutes for exercises with stretching in between exercises, 8-minute jog, and 2-minute cooldown

---

WEEK ONE BOOT CAMP WORKOUT

Monday, Wednesday, Friday:
Resistance Training

1. Warm up.
2. Drink some water.
3. Stretch: standard sequence of fifteen stretches.
4. Twenty-five push-ups: standard, modified, or a combination of both
5. After–push-up stretch: POW stretch (one held thirty seconds)
6. Ten-minute jog or brisk walk
7. Cool down with a walk and water.
8. Bench dips: as many as you can
9. After-dip stretch: left and right triceps stretch (each held ten seconds)
10. Fifty crunches
11. After-crunch stretches: deep breathing and sergeant's salute (one held thirty seconds)
12. Pull-ups: standard, modified, or a combination of both—as many as you can
13. After–pull-up stretches: right and left lat stretches (thirty seconds each); move to upper-back stretches (thirty seconds)
14. Supermen (ten on each side)
15. After-superman stretches: left and right straddle stretches, left and right gluteal stretches, lower-back stretches, and left and right quadriceps stretches (each held thirty seconds)
16. Walk and feel proud.

Come here. Let me look at you. Hey, recruit, do I see a smile on that ugly face of yours?

WEEK ONE BOOT CAMP WORKOUT

Tuesday and Thursday:
Cardio Training

1. Warm up.
2. Stretch.
3. Jog or walk twenty to twenty-five minutes.
4. Cool down.
5. Fifty crunches
6. Twenty supermen

CHAPTER NINE
THE HUMP

Pain is temporary, pride is forever! Now that I have your attention and you can actually move that body, the rest is downhill.

By Week Two, the pants are a little looser, and it's easier to get your rear end out of bed and feel a bit more energized most of the time. As you approach and blast past the hump, you are halfway to the start line. No excuses! I want more results!

> "Hup, down, hup, down," I barked as the class did push-ups. That morning in Boot Camp, Bennie did one too many, even for me. He puked all over his towel. (Give him a break; he could have aimed for someone else's towel.) Fortunately, he was coming up, not going down. Like a good soldier, Bennie just stood up and stretched his pectoral and shoulder muscles.

Are you tired earlier in the day? Seems ironic, yes? You have more energy during Boot Camp and work hours, but you want to go to bed earlier? Listen up for instructions. There could be several reasons why this hits you in Week Two of Boot Camp: Most you can fix with diet; one you can fix by sleeping.

As you go through Boot Camp, you may be tired because of one or even all of the following:

- You're not eating the right foods to sustain your new regimen. Too much sugar in your diet will drag you down.
- You're not eating enough food. This is very common among women first starting an exercise program. You want to see weight

loss and toning results immediately, so you go to extremes with the diet. You need energy to get fit, and you don't have energy without food.

- You're not drinking enough water. Almost everyone falls victim to this at times, even Sargie. Always drink enough water so that your urine is clear—that's an order! I don't mean light yellowish, I mean clear.
- Your tissues are repairing and growing. This is good and normal. You may want to get to bed a little earlier while you are in Boot Camp. You may also want to plan for a nap after your workout to allow your body to recover.

ACHES AND PAINS

Are you sore? Good! If you wear a bra, putting it on should be a challenge. If you wear a sport coat, same thing. It is normal to feel tenderness in the shoulder area from your workout. Try stretching a few minutes before you get dressed to loosen up. (Honestly, if you have to stretch before you dress, you're pretty pathetic.)

After a week in Boot Camp, one of our recruits went to her doctor complaining of chest pain. She said, "I think I'm having a heart attack." He asked her a few questions and did a few tests. Nothing was wrong. He soon learned she had been working out in our fitness program and doing push-ups, pull-ups, and crunches for the first time in her life. At that point, the doctor figured out what her "problem" was and sent her back to Boot Camp.

Do you have pain? Pain is your body's alarm system; listen to it. Here are a few exercises that address pain that is common, but not necessarily a problem.

Shins

Sit on the edge of your chair and play the drums with your toes. Pitter-patter your feet one-hundred times. Very few people actually get shinsplints, but it is common to experience some shin discomfort as you become accustomed to jogging. If you want to jog while you have shin irritation, shuffle your feet as you move.

Neck

Your neck may feel sore from doing abdominal crunches. To relieve it, do a five-part neck stretch before you go to bed: left tilt, right tilt, chin to chest. Don't take this to extremes, though, and try to twist your head like the kid in *The Exorcist*. We do not do neck circles in Boot Camp. I've warned you before: Too much head turning can be hard on your vertebrae.

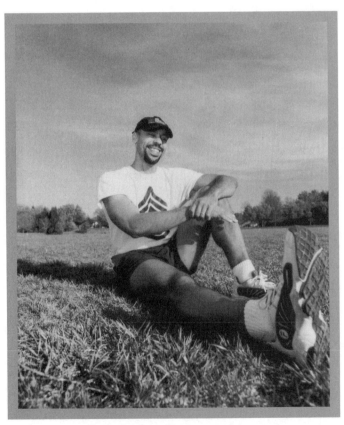

Stretch the hamstrings gently. Ease up if something starts to hurt. And let me see those dentures, recruit!

Hamstrings

The backs of your legs may tingle, or even feel numb, when you try to stretch them. You are pushing too hard if this happens. Ease up on your stretch. Also, be sure you are sitting up straight for the exercise so you don't put extra stress on your back.

In contrast to these types of discomfort, if you feel as if you are being stabbed in the back or shoulders, for example, stop doing the exercise or get a workout partner who doesn't own a knife. (You can count on the Sarge to state the obvious.) See your doctor immediately.

The next thing to remember is: Boot Camp isn't just about exercise. It's about what you put into your body as well as what you do with it.

> Sergeant Ahmad ordered, "Reeeeport!" one morning to his line of recruits. In Boot Camp, "reeeeeport" means "Tell me what you ate yesterday." The first victim he looked at was Charles. Now, being a lawyer, Charles gave a completely honest response. He said, "Um. Not much. I just had some nachos." "Just?" Sergeant Ahmad boomed. "Drop and give me just twenty, Nacho Man!" No one called Charles by his name after that; he was Nacho Man. It helped Charles lose interest in nachos—forever.

Before we go to the workouts for the week, ask yourself if any of the following is a "yes," then check the answers after the test.

1. Nonfat frozen yogurt is as healthy a snack as regular yogurt.
2. Drinking iced tea is as good as drinking water.
3. Low-fat muffins are as good as a bowl of cereal for breakfast.
4. One cookie a day is harmless.
5. A little coffee is fine. It gets you going.

Did you actually say "yes" to any of them? Are you deliberately avoiding the truth or did you just skip chapter 3? Answers and explanations:

1. No. Frozen yogurt has more sweeteners than regular yogurt unless you're buying the wrong kind of regular yogurt. Check your labels: If sugar and corn syrup are high in the list of ingredients, dump the junk down the sink. It amazes me that people think this stuff is a treat. Now hear this, Private Gumby: It is highly likely that frozen yogurt will make you retain water, rot your teeth, and give you gas. And don't give it to your dog. Heaven knows: Dogs (especially Snyper) fart, too.

2. No. Ordinary iced tea contains caffeine; even the herbal and decaffeinated kinds do not clean your body like water. Would you wash your hair with iced tea? Avoid any beverage that has caffeine in it, because it is a diuretic; that is, it pulls water from your body. I spent a good part of chapter 3 telling you how to put water into your body so your insides stay clean and you don't get dehydrated. Don't undo all the good habits you picked up from me by drinking iced tea or those sodas designed to turn us all into caffeine addicts.

3. No. They may be a step up from sugar-encrusted flakes and pops, but they still contain sweeteners and a gum that substitutes for the fat. These muffin turds are a poor substitute for a meal with nutrients; they just take up space so you forget to eat food with value.

4. No. Anything you eat that's extra—that is, it's more than you can use—is not harmless. If you eat anything that boosts your caloric intake beyond what you need, you'll gain weight. A fitness colleague recently told me about research indicating that the average American puts on ten pounds during the winter holidays. That's a lot of cookies going in the mouth . . . one at a time. ("I just had ONE, Sarge!" I know, Elmo, one every ten minutes.) Now don't get me wrong—I know a good cookie when I see one, like oatmeal raisin, but until you get through Boot Camp at least once, no cookies!

5. Welllll, maybe. I hear that coffee enemas do get you going. Trust me, though, this is not what Starbucks or Sargie has in mind.

Sergeant Bill bought thirty-six pounds of chicken fat at the local market and took it to class. He wanted the recruits to find compelling reasons to continue in Boot Camp, so he had each one stick his or her hands in the bag, grab a handful of fat, then put it back in the bag. During the workout they took turns carrying it. He told them, "This is what you're carrying around in your gut, and it'll stay with you the rest of your life if you quit now."

I made it more personal. I put the fat in small plastic bags and had the women put it in their shorts in the back, and the men, under their waistband in the front.

DAY SIX

45-minute workout: 10-minute warm-up, 2-minute cooldown, 8 minutes of stretches, 15 minutes for exercises with stretching in between exercises, 8-minute jog, and 2-minute cooldown

You may want to ask me, "Sarge, how can my workout still be only 45 minutes if I'm doing more push-ups, crunches, dips, pull-ups, and supermen than last week?" You are a bright recruit! The answer has two parts. First, you're better at these exercises than you were last week. Now you can blast out thirty-five push-ups in the same time it took you to drag yourself through twenty-five—I *know* it! Second, you know the workout. When you know what to do next, you go right to it. Good work, boot!

Warm-up

At a slow pace, jog half a mile. Again, as an alternative, you can walk it briskly.

Are you feeling good, alert? Are your eyes straight ahead, glancing down only to stay aware of your terrain? Is your chest out? Are you breathing comfortably and are your hands relaxed? Don't make a fist unless you plan to use it.

Stretches

After you drink some water go straight to your stretches. All of them. It's the most relaxing eight minutes you get in this workout.

Push-ups

You're going to do thirty-five today. Yep, that's ten more than last week. I realize that sometimes people get tired of push-ups. You probably find that hard to believe, because you've done less than a hundred in your life and you can't wait for the next set. For those who become jaded quickly in class, the other sergeants and I have developed ways of making recruits *glad* to do push-ups. Why? They sure as heck don't want to build up muscular strength and endurance by doing this stuff every day:

- Sergeant Lawrence had his Boots push his old, dingy gray, nasty-smelling, Fred Flintstone Ford Fiesta down the street. (He still has this car.)
- Sergeant Bill ordered recruits in his class to push picnic tables around the park. Picnic table races usually bang up the shins, but they're good for spirit.
- I made one slacker getting ready to enter ROTC go with me to a construction site. I had him pick up cinder blocks and move them from one pile to another while I barked orders. All the construction workers gathered around and laughed at him; their big guts were bouncing up and down. When he got the whole pile done, I yelled, "What's this pile doing here? Pick 'em up and move 'em back over there!"

How many push-ups should you do today? Sergeant Dick, a native of a war-torn country, has the formula. Alleging that his ability to count in English isn't very good, he bases the number on the world news. If there is an uprising in Sierra Leone that kills eighty-two people, that's the count for the day. If the stock market was up forty-two points yesterday, maybe that's the target. For the people in his class, the morning paper takes on a new meaning.

I'm going to offer you an alternative, too. Instead of doing push-ups today, how would you like to rearrange all the furniture in your house? No? Then get down! Nose, nipples, navel—report for duty!

After-Push-up Stretch

The POW stretch feels sooo good.

Jog or Brisk Walk

Time for your fifteen-minute run or power walk. Don't feel like it? I know how to excite people like you: I take them mountain climbing. MY version of mountain climbing is running uphill on gravel, which actually means you're not running anywhere. It's like a treadmill. Fun, huh? (Don't try this without me, recruit. This is an advanced move.)

Cooldown

Where's your water bottle?

Doing a mile-long jog without a cooldown is hard on your body. When you're out there storming the streets with your chest out and nostrils flaring, your heart is pumping and blood is racing to your muscles. If you just stop cold, you don't give the blood flow a chance to slow down. I've told you before and I'll tell you again: This could make you dizzy, or you could faint or puke. So if you want to skip the cooldown, you better stand near your blanket and don't come near me.

Dips

Do as many as you can—twice. After you do the first set, you will need to rest. Use this minute or two to breathe, drink some water, and stretch. When you hit the bench again, imagine yourself with powerful arms. Think about pointing, or raising your arm to reach for something and knowing that the back of your arm is firm, not flapping like a turkey neck. Arrrgggghhh! You can do it, reeeecruit!

After-Dip Stretch

Left and right triceps stretch (each one held ten seconds).

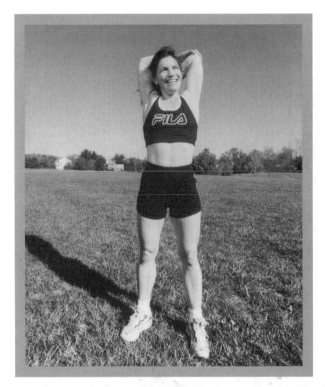

After two tough sets of dips, you should be happy to do this stretch if your deodorant's working.

Crunches

This week, you WILL aim for sixty.

After-Crunch Stretches

Remember to breathe deeply while you're on your back, then go straight to the sergeant's salute (one held thirty seconds).

Pull-ups

You are so lucky! You get to do two sets this week. Do the kind of pull-up that you can manage for about fifteen repetitions. Take a short break and, just like the break between bench dips, use the time to breathe, drink some water, and stretch. After that, hit the bar again and do as many as you can.

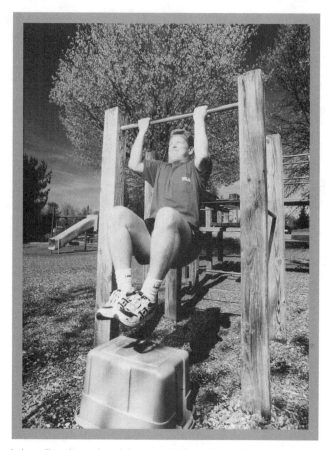

He's doing fine keeping his negative pull-up slow, but if he doesn't breathe, he'll bust a hemorrhoid . . . and I hate that.

After-Pull-up Stretches

Go straight from your latissimus dorsi stretches (thirty seconds each) to the upper-back stretch, with fingertips together in front of you and your head down (thirty seconds).

The Superman

Last week, I wanted ten on each side. This week, I don't ask for much more—just twelve.

After-Superman Stretches

Good work, recruit, you're almost done. After straddle stretches, gluteal stretches, the lower-back stretch, and quadriceps stretches,

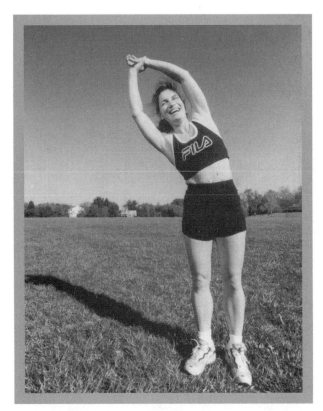

After this fun move, stand up straight, drop your arms and head
forward and stretch your upper back.

you can drink some water, take a short walk, and get your nice,
firm butt to the office.

Congratulations—you've begun another great week!

DAYS SEVEN AND NINE

45-minute workout: 5-minute warm-up, 2-minute cooldown, 8
minutes of stretches, 20-minute aerobic
workout, 5-minute cooldown, 5 minutes of
crunches and supermen

Warm-up

Take the usual five minutes to tiptoe through the wet grass, then
have a couple ounces of water.

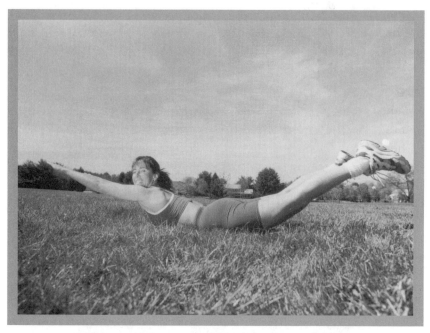

Some people really think they're Superman when they do this
exercise. I think they look more like Jimmy Olsen.

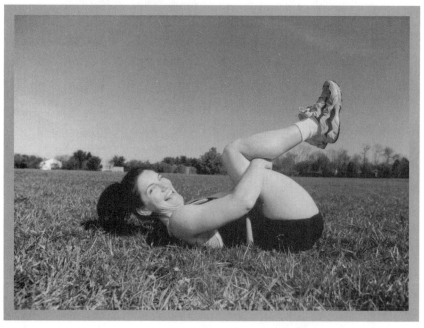

No one forgets the Sergeant's Salute.

Stretches

Check the last chapter if you have not memorized the sequence and do twenty penalty push-ups for being lazy.

Jog

Take twenty to twenty-five minutes for your run or power walk. If you take my advice on breathing, this will not seem like an eternity in hell. Remember that deep breathing is out. Breathing in four stages is your goal: in (first half breath), in (final half breath), out (first half of exhale), out (final half). These are small breaths that happen every time your foot strikes the ground.

Cooldown

Walk around proudly and slowly like a filly (or a stallion) that's just won the Kentucky Derby. Drink water.

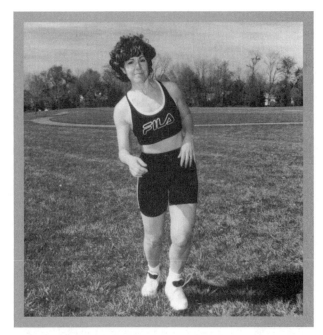

You'll look like this after 20 minutes if you don't stand up straight and breathe right.

Crunches

What did you do yesterday? Sixty crunches? Hah! Not today! On Day Seven you do *two sets of fifty.* Yes, you can take a break between them. And what do you do during your rest breaks—lie on the grass with your tongue hanging out? Not MY recruits! You drink water, stretch, and visualize how tight your gut is getting.

The Superman

Just like Day Six, you aim for twenty-four.

> Midway through his second week in Boot Camp, Dr. Z admitted, "I'm still stressed out from my work, but at least I have more energy while I'm feeling my stress."

DAYS EIGHT AND TEN

45-minute workout: 10-minute warm-up, 2-minute cooldown, 8 minutes of stretches, 15 minutes for exercises with stretching in between exercises, 8-minute jog, and 2-minute cooldown

Can you remember what you did on Monday? I'll remind you at the end of the chapter.

> Gerald had come back to Boot Camp after falling off the food wagon. A former graduate of the program, he let life overwhelm him for a couple years. In that time, he gained sixty pounds and started smoking. During the mile run on the first day in Boot Camp—which for him was a walk—Gerald repeatedly coughed up what Sergeant Ahmad called "green glue." "That's the sticky stuff that's kept your lungs from working. Hack it up and get it over with, soldier!" he barked. That day, Gerald did a couple push-ups on his knees.

Eight days into the program—and this included what he called a "terrible weekend of fat-man food"—Gerald ran the entire mile and was able to do ten push-ups on his toes. Clean living on the other days had also helped him lose eight pounds.

"I look forward to getting up in the morning," he said. "And even though I feel like I can't do much while I'm at Boot Camp, by the afternoon, I feel like I can do anything—like I could run ten miles. That feeling keeps me high, and it makes me anticipate going back to exercise the next day."

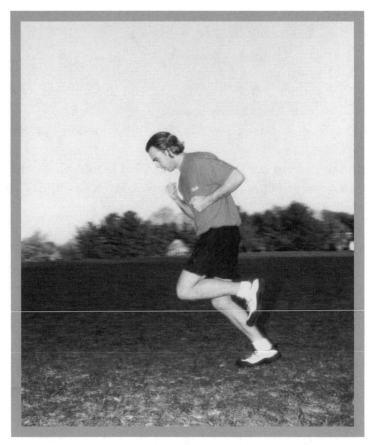

If you look like this, straighten up and slow down to a walk.

WEEK TWO BOOT CAMP WORKOUT

Monday, Wednesday, Friday
Resistance Training

1. Warm up.
2. Drink some water.
3. Stretch: standard sequence of fifteen stretches
4. Thirty-five pushups: standard, modified, or a combination of both
5. After–push-up stretch: POW stretch (one held thirty seconds)
6. Fifteen-minute jog or brisk walk
7. Cool down with a walk and water.
8. Bench dips: as many as you can—twice
9. After-dip stretch: left and right triceps stretch (each held ten seconds)
10. Sixty crunches
11. After-crunch stretches: deep breathing and sergeant's salute (one held thirty seconds)
12. Pull-ups: standard, modified, or a combination—twice; do as many as you can.
13. After–pull-up stretches: right and left lat stretches (thirty seconds each); move to upper-back stretches (thirty seconds).
14. Twenty-four supermen (twelve on each side)
15. After-superman stretches: left/right straddle stretches, left/right gluteal stretches, lower-back stretches, and left/right quad stretches (each held thirty seconds)
16. Walk and feel proud.

WEEK TWO BOOT CAMP WORKOUT

Tuesday and Thursday:

Cardio Training

1. Warm up.
2. Stretch.
3. Jog or walk twenty to twenty-five minutes.
4. Cool down.
5. Crunches: two sets of fifty each
6. Twenty-five supermen

CHAPTER TEN
READY FOR A STRIPE

Pull your bootstraps up: Week Three is tough, but you've come a long way and you can go all the way! Just like the past two weeks, I'm going to give you a pat on the back and a kick in the ass every day.

> The second time our fitness program ever got publicity, the local newspaper covered the Boot Camp final test. "Don't do anything screwy," I told the class, which was all male. "I want you in short haircuts, clean-shaven, and ready to move." Every one of them showed up in Hawaiian shirts and leis. One guy brought his dog.

This week, you are preparing for your final test, administered on the last day of Boot Camp, which tells me whether or not you can graduate to a more challenging maintenance program. If you don't pass it, you will repeat Boot Camp. Join the crowd: Forty percent of everyone who completes Boot Camp gets to repeat; that does *not* mean you are a failure. This is not a pass-fail situation; it's a starting point on your road to fitness.

In fact, if you are one of the many people who will go through Boot Camp again, you'll find it more fun the second or third time around simply because you know what you're doing and are more capable than the first time. You are moving toward greater fitness and confidence in your body.

DAYS ELEVEN, THIRTEEN, AND FIFTEEN

45-minute workout: 10-minute warm-up, 2-minute cooldown,
8 minutes of stretches, 15 minutes for exercises with stretching in between exercises,
8-minute jog, and 2-minute cooldown

For most of you, this means Monday, Wednesday, and Friday. You won't notice much difference between this week and last in terms of what you do, but you will notice a *big* difference in how you feel: You are so much stronger by this time that "two sets of maximum" dips and pull-ups will be more than last week, and you will do more push-ups on your toes than before.

Here's the drill:

After your five-minute warm-up, drink a little water, then do your eight minutes of blissful stretches. When you do your set of forty-five push-ups, do as many as you can at the highest difficulty level you have achieved. If that means on the deck, then go from your toes to your knees when you get tired. If you began on your knees, that might mean you'll have to finish up by pushing off a bench. I know I don't have to tell you to stretch after each exercise, right, tough guy? After your stretch, go straight to the fifteen-minute jog, then turn it into a walk so you can slow down and drink your water without spilling it. Finish up two sets of dips to the maximum, seventy crunches, two smokin' sets of pull-ups, thirty supermen, and a long soak in the hot tub, or if you're from the East Coast, a hot shower.

The summary is waiting for you just before the instructions on your test. I do make things easy for you, don't I?

DAYS TWELVE AND FOURTEEN

45-minute workout: 5-minute warm-up, 2-minute cooldown,
8 minutes of stretches, 20-minute aerobic
workout, 5-minute cooldown, 5 minutes of
crunches and supermen

Since Tuesdays and Thursdays are your hard-charging cardio days, after you warm up and stretch, head out for your twenty- to twenty-five-minute jog or very brisk walk. Cool down, then move straight to three sets of fifty crunches. Squeeeeze those abs—make this count! Finish up with a set of thirty supermen.

Again, the summary for your cardio workout is later in this chapter.

Let's have a quiz, now that you think you have this whole routine under control and know everything there is to know about fitness. Remember when you were a kid—quizzes were always ten questions. Ten little things you didn't know beans about unless you actually paid attention in class, and that only happened when you thought you might flunk. Well, reeecruit, this time teacher is a real hard-ass:

1. Why do I tell you to stretch after each exercise?
2. How are you supposed to breathe when you jog or walk briskly?
3. Why is it so important to cool down after you exercise hard?
4. Why should you drink water while you exercise?
5. Why do you do resistance exercises like push-ups (arrrggghhh, give me twenty!)?
6. How hard should you exercise at any given time in Boot Camp?
7. What are good sources of water other than water (this is not a trick question)?
8. How much muscle does a slacker lose every year?
9. What do you always do before you jog?
10. Who can you count on to kick your butt and hold your hand at the same time?

Bonus question: How many pounds of fat did Gerald put on after he quit Boot Camp?

Ten correct answers gets you a smile from your good-lookin' Sarge. Get the bonus question correct, and Gerald will remain pissed at me.

For every wrong answer, you give me five penalty push-ups. If you get number ten wrong, give me fifty, jerky! The answers are right here:

1. Any time you contract a muscle, you need to re-lengthen it. Skip your stretches and you are asking—I mean, begging—for

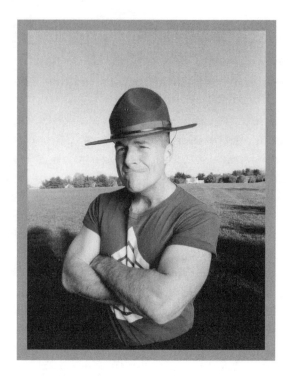

injury and soreness. The first thing you're going to want to skip is stretching because you're stiff, and that is back assward from what you need to be doing. Stretching is extra important. Don't blow it off.

I've seen macho recruits go all out with their pull-ups and push-ups and crunches so they can be babe magnets by the end of Boot Camp, then when it comes time to stretch, you'd think I had asked them to sweep the floor with their tongues. They are not your role models—I am.

2. When you jog or walk briskly always do a four-part breath: in (step)-in (step), out (step)-out (step) with your mouth slightly puckered as if you are going to whistle. Keep a cadence like the one in chapter 8 going in your head. The rhythm will help regulate your breathing.

3. Remember why it is so important to cool down after a hard workout? Is it something about feeling dizzy, fainting, or throwing up on your lawn if you don't?

4. Water lubricates your joints and maintains your body's tem-

perature. Be smart about this: You need to drink a few ounces every ten or fifteen minutes whether it's hot or cold outside. Without sufficient water, you will feel dizzy and fatigued.

5. You do resistance exercises to build muscle strength and endurance. Strength is the ability to move an object once; endurance is the ability to move it repeatedly. A pull-up is your ability to lift your lard ass off the ground. Five pull-ups means you have the endurance to pass at least part of your Boot Camp test.

6. Stay within the twelve to sixteen range of the Perceived Exertion chart in Boot Camp. That's somewhere between starting to sweat and stinking like a teenage boy's locker. Anytime you feel out of breath, throttle it back.

7. Fresh juice, fruits, and vegetables are good sources of water. Beer is not juice.

8. Loafers lose half a pound of muscle a year. You must DO something to stop that muscle loss or you will get progressively more like a bowl of Jell-O. Once you start exercising—like in Boot Camp—you are on the way to regaining what you lost.

9. Before you jog, you must catch up on the world news or read your favorite book as you enjoy a Sergeant's Private Moment.

10. Puleeeeeze don't tell me you need help on this one!

Answer to the bonus question: Gerald added sixty pounds to his flabby, hairy, I-can-no-longer-see-my-peepee stomach. But he's back in action now and promises—to himself mostly, and that's what counts—that he will never let that happen again. He respects himself and he's having a blast. Way to go, Gerald! You're the man!

Are you ready for your Boot Camp test? Not yet? Here's some inspiration.

• Three years after they completed Boot Camp, The Welsh Park Buttnuts, a group of fifteen graduates who continued to exercise together, competed in a marathon—successfully. The same group also travels to Colorado on a week-long ski trip every year.

• A sixty-two-year-old woman came to Boot Camp with one goal:

to focus her mind on something positive and get some blessed relief from her stress. At the time, her husband was dying of cancer and she was caring for a brain-damaged grandchild. She made it!

• Every year, we sponsor a Jolly Fat Man's Run: seven miles through some of the most scenic parts of Washington, D.C., and a nearby suburb. It's just before the Christmas holiday, so every Boot Camp grad in the run gets a reminder of the rewards of saying "HECK NO!" to Grandma's cookies. The first year, we had fifty people. In 1997, the number grew to eighty-five— some run and some walk the seven miles. One of our walkers was a man who had graduated from Boot Camp five months prior to the event. When he entered the program, he was 150 pounds overweight. By the time he did the run, he was down to seventy-five pounds overweight. He finished *and* he's still losing weight!

THE TEST

Calm down, you silly freak! Take the test, then if you don't like the results, just take it again. In fact, if you spend the next six months taking this test every day, you'll be on the fast track to fitness.

In order to graduate, you must have a passing performance in at least three of the five areas. If you earn a bonus in one area, you can use it to cancel a low grade in another area. Hear me, though: You can only count bonuses in two areas.

I respect the fact that you may have made great progress but are still not ready to pull your full weight in a pull-up or do every push-up on your toes. You can still pass this test by doing modified versions of both those exercises.

	Passing	Bonus
Push-ups	50	60
Mile	10:00	9:00
Bench dips	25	35
Crunches	100	125
Pull-ups	5	7

WEEK THREE BOOT CAMP WORKOUT

Monday, Wednesday, Friday:
Resistance Training

1. Warm up.
2. Drink some water.
3. Stretch: standard sequence of fifteen stretches.
4. Forty-five push-ups: standard, modified, or a combination of both
5. After–pushup stretch: POW stretch (one held thirty seconds).
6. Fifteen-minute jog or brisk walk
7. Cool down with a walk and water.
8. Bench dips: as many as you can—twice
9. After-dip stretch: left and right triceps stretch (each held ten seconds)
10. Seventy crunches
11. After-crunch stretches: deep breathing and sergeant's salute (one held thirty seconds)
12. Pull-ups: standard, modified, or a combination—twice; do as many as you can.
13. After–pull-up stretches: right and left lat stretches (thirty seconds each); move to upper-back stretches (thirty seconds)
14. Thirty supermen (fifteen on each side)
15. After-superman stretches: left and right straddle stretches, left and right gluteal stretches, lower-back stretches, and left and right quadriceps stretches (each held thirty seconds)
16. Satisfaction

> ## WEEK THREE BOOT CAMP WORKOUT
>
> Tuesday and Thursday:
> Cardio Training
>
> 1. Warm up.
> 2. Stretch.
> 3. Jog or walk twenty to twenty-five minutes.
> 4. Cool down.
> 5. Crunches: three sets of fifty each
> 6. Thirty supermen
> 7. Shout Hoooraahhh!

Push-ups

As soon as you can no longer do them in perfect form on your toes, drop to your knees. I don't want your back sagging like an old nag and your gut dragging on the ground. If and when you drop to your knees, keep them close together. I've seen recruits spread their knees out so far, I thought they'd split in half. Doing modified push-ups in that position will NOT earn you bonus points.

The Mile

Remember: This is fun. Gasping for air is not fun, so slow down and enjoy the view for your mile, even it means you walk most of it. You will get faster over time. If you push yourself too hard, you'll impress no one but the mortician.

Bench Dips

If these are now so easy for you that you can pump out more than the bonus number, you are ready to graduate to bar dips using your full body weight. Congratulations! I'll teach you those in the next chapter.

Crunches

Really contract your abs, even though it's a test and you want to knock out a quick hundred. Just lifting your head off the ground—what I call a neck-up—is not passing form.

Pull-ups

You can substitute fifteen modified pull-ups, or twenty-five for the bonus, for the standard full-body-weight version. Use a bar that is about waist high and rest your feet on the ground. The more you bend your knees, the easier this is, so try to start out with your legs straight then move to a bent-knee position.

Log your results. We're not done yet, so hang on to your pencil.

Grab your seamstress tape measure—the one you put in a bathroom drawer after you took your initial measurements.

- Record your height in inches. If it's different from the measurement you took three weeks ago, I'd like to know about it and so would your tailor.
- Men and women, have someone help you measure your neck and abdominal area. Refer to chapter 2 if you forgot how. Take each measurement twice and record the average. Women only: In addition to measuring your neck and ab areas, also record your hip measurement. Use the body-fat grid in Appendix A again to determine your body composition. Men, subtract your neck measurement from your waist measurement, then refer to the grid to get an approximation of your percentage of body fat. Women, add your waist and hip measurements, then subtract the circumference of your neck and refer to the grid. Log the number.
- Optional: Weigh yourself and record the result. Keep in mind that muscle weighs more than fat, so the tape measure will help you understand the changes in your body more than the scale. If you are one of those people who feels motivated toward fitness by losing weight, then by all means, weigh yourself. Just don't make this the most important or, worse yet, the only measure of your progress.

Here is the activity that's far more important than the test: Contrast the results of your Boot Camp final test and your new body measurements with the numbers you logged three weeks ago.

Even slight progress—the loss of an inch around your waist, or the ability to do a couple extra push-ups or jog a mile in twelve minutes instead of thirteen—is a huge accomplishment. I want to shake your hand!

An overweight salesman showed up one morning with a big grin on his face. One of his fellow recruits asked, "What's up? You look pretty happy." The man replied, "I've lost 125 pounds since I started this program." "You can't be serious!" "Yeah, man. My divorce just went through."

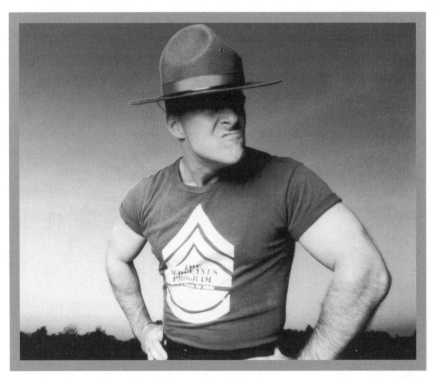

You want reasons to keep exercising? LISTEN UP!

CHAPTER ELEVEN

WHAT NOW, SARGE?

Dying is easy. It's living that scares me to death.

Annie Lennox

Take a deep breath and let it out. Fill your lungs with air, then exhale very slowly. Feel good? You are about to feel better. I am going to do two things for you: Fill your head with facts about the great things you are doing for your body, mind, and spirit—things that make living an experience you *enjoy*—and introduce you to "graduate level" exercises.

Of course, along with the good news, I'll also tell you what will happen if you stop exercising. Why? I want you to take action every day to avoid backsliding. You may consider Boot Camp over if you passed your test, but Boot Camp is just an introduction, a way to get the momentum going. Your road to fitness has just begun. Now that you have surprised yourself by moving from a walk to a jog, pumping out a few push-ups, and trimming some fat off your lard butt, keep moving forward. Keep having fun!

Let's say you gained strength at the rate of 5 percent a week during Boot Camp. That's not outrageous by any means; your quickest cycle of fitness is in the first ninety days of an exercise program. In fact, the elderly people in the study I talked about in chapter 6 tripled their strength in only eight weeks and had a 16 percent muscle tissue growth. Because you see the greatest results in this initial period, you will probably push the hardest and be more daring than at any other time. You'll buy some new pants with a smaller waist, flash a toothy grin when your friends tell you how wonderful you look, and offer to help your spouse clean out the stinking garage. Imagine how strong, vigorous, brave, courageous, bold you will be if you just repeat Boot Camp three times in these ninety days. You'll have to bolt your door to stop Jerry Maguire from hounding you for a contract!

What if you decide to "take a break" now because you can do a handful of pull-ups and you've lost ten pounds of middle-age flab? You know you are better off than before, so you might get lulled into complacency. Here's a happy fact about your progress that can come back to bite you in the ass: If you gained strength at the rate of 5 percent a week, you will lose it only at the rate of about 2½ percent a week, because strength loss occurs at half the rate of gain. "Not so bad," you say? "I'll just pick up this book and start all over when all the gains are gone." DON'T BE A BONE-HEAD—there's another factor that takes effect quickly and immediately.

If you eat the same when you stop exercising as you did when you were smokin' yourself in Boot Camp, all those calories that used to help you get through your workout have no place to go but to your hips, your middle, and wherever else you store lard. You may protest, "I'm still eating clean, Sarge!" After I congratulate you, I'll also kick you in the rear end for not getting the message: Any calories you take in beyond those you can use will cause a weight gain. You have to work them off, buttnut!

There is a list of 5,790.2 additional health reasons why you should continue to exercise. I don't want to insult your intelligence by naming them all, but I will highlight the extreeeeemely important ones. First of all, let me give you a big pat on the back for taking action to prevent heart disease, injuries from doing everyday things, humpback from osteoporosis, body fat, bad cholesterol (LDL), high blood pressure, and a lousy attitude.

Exercise decreases your risk of all these nasty conditions. Listen to me: The reason exercise has this effect is because it impacts your body *systems*, not just your body shape. Please don't leave Boot Camp behind like you left summer camp as a kid. Memories of feeling fit don't keep you fit!

After President Eisenhower survived a heart attack during his first term in office (for you youngsters like me, that was in the mid-

1950s), the country became more aware of the need to prevent heart attacks. Studies about this flourished. One of them revealed that the only inner-city population that did not have a problem with heart attacks was the longshoremen. The reason, despite their less-than-perfect diet, was that their daily lives involved strenuous labor. By exerting themselves at high levels for twenty, thirty, or forty years every day, they prevented heart disease.

> During a visit to one of the program's corporate clients, I went in to see the employee benefits director. She was bragging about the fact that, over the past five weeks, she had dropped sixteen pounds through some popular diet. No exercise, just diet. I looked around her office: a printer, computer, copier, water cooler, scale, file cabinet, phone with an intercom, coffeemaker. In short, she didn't have to leave the office except to go to the bathroom and go home! After five years in this office, of course she needed a fat-loss program. I got her away from the killer conveniences, and she got smart and started parking on the far side of the employee lot. *Now* she's making progress.

You may find that the greatest rewards of exercise are not even physical ones, and that the 5,790.2 facts about disease and injury prevention don't move you one bit. I have seen many, many cases where the unexpected psychoemotional rewards top all the others: feeling like a kid, not getting aggravated by rain or snow, anticipating being awake instead of going to sleep. A sense of fun starts with feeling good.

Here are some of the things Boots have said to me about working out in Boot Camp. And you'd better believe their sense of fun and accomplishment carries over to their professions and their personal lives.

- A thirty-five-year-old CPA: "This is the only thing (besides sex, of course) that can get me up at 5 A.M. with a smile on my face."

- A thirty-five-year-old lawyer: "We did push-ups, stomach crunches—all in the mud. I thought it was a great experience."
- A forty-four-year-old insurance salesman: "I feel like I can do anything . . . exercising keeps me high."

Exercise is an eye-opener in lots of ways, isn't it?

One morning—this actually describes more than one—I had a group of professional women in a class outside at 6 A.M. It was thirty-eight degrees and the sun had no chance of shining. As we started our exercises, the rain came. Not a word of complaint. I don't want you to think I had them scared or intimidated, either. Do you think the Sarge would threaten to maim anyone who didn't co-operate? No, they were moving their bodies; that's what helped them have a positive spirit. They were wet and muddy and laughing. When was the last time you put those three experiences all together? Hopefully, at least once over the past three weeks.

Beyond the shift in attitude that Boot Camp can help you make, another reward to lift your spirits is how you look. I'm not going to pretend that's not important; that's probably why you picked up this book in the first place. There are a few angles to the reward that you may not have considered, though.

First, the attitude about yourself that you project affects how others react to you. Haven't you noticed that, on days when you feel energetic and happy, people are more likely to compliment you on your appearance? You might have heard it a lot over these past three weeks. You may not have changed your shape more than a centimeter at the thighs or love handles, but you still project a better self-image. What people see is what you feel!

Men, save yourself a trip to the hair plug store: Keep exercising!

Women, get your check back from the boob doctor: Keep exercising!

When they first come to Boot Camp, a lot of women look older than they are; they are the moms, literally or figuratively. They care for and nurture people around them—their coworkers and their kids—and spend very little time on themselves, except to cover up the dark circles under their eyes with makeup. They bear the burden of the family's well-being on their own shoulders and don't give a thought to self-preservation. By coming to Boot Camp, they finally do something more meaningful for themselves than get their gray hair dyed, and the results are magnificent. You're supposed to care for yourself, recruits! Mom, put some low-fat milk, cereal, and fruit out for the kids and run out the door to do your workout before you run off to the office! You'll look ten years younger in a couple of months.

I'm really good at guessing ages, but one women who came to Boot Camp completely surprised me. When I asked for her age, I thought she was in her late 40s. Nope. She was my age—that's ten years younger. Fortunately, I didn't throw a number at her. Sure enough, she had gone through a lot of stress in her life, with her husband declaring bankruptcy and the family depending on her to be the breadwinner. Each day in the program did more for her appearance than any $90 cream could ever do.

Compare pictures of yourself—just your face—before and during Boot Camp. You'll see exactly what I mean.

In the past couple of years, I've seen more and more women go through Boot Camp. These women are among the many who will redefine what looking your age means, so at some point, "looking fifty" will translate to "having a youthful appearance" not "approaching saggy and baggy."

Does this only apply to women? No, jerky! Take the Sarge as an example. I happen to look better than I did when I was a teenager in the Navy, except I had more hair then, and my stamina is better than a teenager's. Ask my wife.

If one of the rewards you have experienced is the satisfaction of passing the test, hoooraahhh! It is important to challenge yourself to continue to progress, so you may want to move on to the next level. I warn you, though. Don't try anything beyond Boot Camp if you did not legitimately pass the test! The other exercises are more difficult, and you might hurt yourself. If your partner passed and you didn't, get another Boot Camp buddy. Let your friend move on now and join him or her later.

BEYOND BOOT CAMP

Here are techniques to transition from Boot Camp to a tougher fitness routine that you can use to maintain and gain endurance and strength. Remember: *Always* do your stretches in the pre-scribed order during your routine! Don't become "muscle bound" by focusing exclusively on your strength-building exercises.

LISTEN UP!

Use only the workout intensity techniques that apply to you. If you did not meet the minimum test requirement in a category, your goal should be to meet that before you make the exercise more difficult.

Push-ups

Over the next few weeks, you will challenge your muscles in a slightly different way by doing push-ups more slowly on some days, adding reps on others, and trying to do longer sets.

Doing push-ups slowly gives you "time in tension." This will stress your muscles to the point of increased blood flow and, in turn, strengthen the muscle fibers you recruit for the exercise. Aim for a four-second push-up: down for a slow count of two and up for a slow two. You may find this method is hard as heck; but do it, Mighty Mouse, and you will get stronger! Just keep your body aligned properly to avoid back strain.

Your Week Three target was forty-five, so stay with that in Week Four, but do them to the four-count. If it takes you three sets of fif-teen to do forty-five quality push-ups in Week Four, shoot for two sets—a set of twenty-five and a set of twenty—in Week Five. Week Six, see how many fast push-ups you can do in one set, then rest, stretch, and do another set to exhaustion. Week Seven set a higher target, like fifty, and do them at a slow pace in three sets. Reduce that to two sets of twenty-five in Week Eight, and so on.

Dips

If you did bench dips with ease, you are ready for bar dips.

Find strong bars that are a little more than shoulder-width apart. Start with your arms fully extended, but not locked. Slowly lower your body until the elbows are flexed at ninety degrees or the upper arms are parallel to the floor. Slowly press your body back to the start position. Repeat this as many times as you can. Again, the count of two seconds up and two down defines "slowly." Be sure you do not drop down quickly or go too deep. Doing that will place too much stress on your shoulders and chest muscles. Increase the repetitions using the same weekly schedule you stuck to when doing bench dips in Boot Camp.

Pull-ups

If you exceeded the bonus number of seven standard pull-ups on your Boot Camp test, Hoooraahhh! You are one in a million—most kids can't even do that! Every week, just add a couple more to get stronger. You could also try a slightly wider grip. Bodybuilders use it to work the upper-back muscles hard to get that V-shape from the shoulders to the waist.

Good luck with doing four-second pull-ups—they even make Sargie sweat—but I do recommend keeping them as slow as possible. The last thing you want is a joint dislocation or tendinitis from doing pull-ups too darned fast.

Crunches

Do them more slowly, squeezing as you contract. Believe me, you can make one-hundred crunches very, very challenging this way, and your abdominal muscles will serve you well.

Supermen

Since this exercise works your lower back, remember to increase level of difficulty with it as you make your crunches tougher. Your abs and your lower-back muscles work together to hold you erect, and you need to keep them in balance.

Don't go nuts with this exercise, though: Never do more than forty repetitions at one time or you'll have a hard time standing up.

Running

Here are three ways to pump up your cardiorespiratory workouts on Tuesdays and Thursdays:

1. Increase the amount of time you run rather than walk, until you can run the entire mile.
2. Add two minutes to your run on cardio days, then keep increasing a little at a time, but never add more than ten percent per week of running time or distance. If you ran a total of ten miles last week, this week add only one mile. If you choose to ignore me on this one, go ahead, call your local orthopedic surgeon right now for an appointment, 'cause you'll need it.
3. Add a small hill to your run.

Steve lost fifty pounds in the time he went through Boot Camp and began regularly coming to Maintenance Program workouts. He said, "The day I don't show, call the police or the hospital. I'm either dead or sick." He never missed a class for an entire year. One day he didn't show up, so I got concerned. He was in the hospital with acute gall bladder trouble.

Are there actually a few of you reading this book who haven't done anything yet? Did you just pick it up to laugh at how many times I use the word "butt"? You're crazy! The purpose of this book is to be entertaining while you exercise. You receive no benefit, other than insight into my personality, unless you *use* the stuff in this book. Sarge says: Knowledge not applied is worthless!

As for the rest of you who learned to enjoy the process of fitness, think of Jimmy Stewart in *It's a Wonderful Life*. He got another chance to live. So did you.

A NOTE TO MOM

My Dearest Mother,

I know you taught me to use much nicer words than the ones in this book. Please understand that it is my mission to move poor, misguided souls toward a life of better health and well-being, and using these words is part of how I do that. Anyway, yell at Dad. He's the one who taught me the bad words.

With love and innocence,
Sarge

DEFINITIONS OF BOOT CAMP WORDS AND OTHER IMPORTANT FITNESS TERMS

Abduction—Movement away from the body (like a stinky). When you lift your arms to reach a pull-up bar, you abduct them.

Adduction—Movement toward your body. It's the opposite of abduction.

Adipose tissue—Fat, as in "your ass."

Aerobic—With oxygen, or in the presence of oxygen.

Aerobic endurance—Ability to jog with Sarge screaming at you.

Aerobic exercise—The morning jog you do in Boot Camp. Not to be confused with leotard dancing.

Amino acids—Building blocks of protein. If you don't have a balanced diet, you don't get all the amino acids you need to survive Boot Camp.

Anaerobic—opposite of aerobic, so it means "without oxygen," or "without the presence of oxygen."

Anaerobic training—Strength training is essentially anaerobic. That does not mean you don't breathe.

Arteries—Large blood vessels that carry oxygenated blood away from the heart to the tissues. Don't clog them with fat, or oxygenated blood can't get to the heart. We call that a heart attack waiting to happen.

Arthritis—Inflammation of the joints. Not fun.

Atrophy— Shrinking muscle. See also "worthless bag of atrophy."

Blood pooling—A condition generally caused by vigorous exercise ending quickly. Your blood moves away from the brain, so you may feel light-headed. If this happens, sit your behind down and call room service because you are going to stay there for a while. Remember why I told you to cool down after you jog? Next time listen, my pale-faced parsnip!

Blood pressure—Pressure of blood in arteries. A normal reading is around 120/80; if you're really fit, it's lower. If it's higher, you may be hypertensive, i.e., you have high blood pressure. Also see "systolic" and "diastolic."

Body-fat measurement—There are several ways to measure your body fat: skinfold measurements done with calipers, electrical impedance (sounds shocking), infrared, underwater weighing, and the approximation we do with body measurements and a grid. Some are more accurate than others. The grid method used for Boot Camp is roughly 3 percent off; so are a couple of the others. Most important, use the same device each time so you have a consistent point of reference.

Brown fat—Don't worry about it; found within muscle tissue. You have to realize that every time we say "fat," we don't necessarily mean something bad. Fat insulates the body, contributes to cellular health, and is a source of energy.

Bursa—Fluid-filled sac located at points of pressure; it alleviates friction in joints.

Bursitis—Inflammation of the bursa; this is what happens when you abuse your joints.

Buttnut—One who doesn't listen well.

CPR—Cardiopulmonary resuscitation; what you will hope someone else can do if you didn't follow the instructions in this book.

Calorie—A unit of energy; it is also what you may have eaten too many of. One gram of fat gives you nine calories, one gram of carbohydrate or protein gives you four.

Carbohydrate—Food generally found, not raised, in a garden or pasture, but there are exceptions, such as pasta. Personally, I have never seen linguini in a freshly fertilized field.

Cardiovascular exercise—What you need thirty minutes of at least a couple days a week—walk, jog, run, swim.

Chronic—Describes a condition that persists over time, as in, "A lazy recruit causes a chronic pain in the hip for Sarge."

Concentric contraction—Otherwise known as the "positive" when exerting: when pulling yourself up to the pull-up bar, when you're crunching the crunch, pushing up from a dip, pushing up in a push-up.

Cookie monster—One who is snack-challenged.

Diabetes—A disease in which the body won't metabolize carbohydrates normally.

Diastolic pressure—Blood pressure in arteries when the heart relaxes between contractions. It's the lower number in 120/80. Also, see "systolic."

Diaphram—Rubber device inserted just before . . . just kidding. It's a domelike sheet of muscle responsible for contracting during breathing. A "side stitch" when you jog means lack of oxygen to that area.

Diuretic—A substance, like caffeine, that increases renal excretion. In other words, it makes you pee a lot.

Dough boy—One who is in the program, but refuses to make an effort to lose weight. See buttnut.

Eccentric contraction—Otherwise known as "the negative" part of an exercise. This is the contraction that happens when you slowly lower yourself from a pull-up or a push-up.

Ectomorph—A long, skinny body type, like a lot of fourteen-year-old basketball players.

Edema—Swelling, or excessive body fluid in tissues. You might see this if you overtax a joint, so don't.

Empty calories—The kind of calories you get from food and drink with no nutritional value, like those white cake things with nasty frosting that kids want in their lunch boxes, or a shot of bourbon.

Endomorph—Heavy body type (hint: *d* is a fat letter). It's tough for folks like this to keep fat off, but it's not impossible. No excuses!

Endorphin—A natural hormone that produces pain-inhibiting qualities. It's the feel-good hormone found during exercise; it's what causes that "natural high" that helps marathon runners smile for pictures at mile twenty-six.

Enzyme—Proteins that cause certain chemical changes in the body. You need them to turn food into energy.

Ergogenic aid—Something that helps you to improve strength or endurance, like sneakers. Actually, that's a stretch. It usually refers to substances like dietary supplements and steriods, energy bars, and carb drinks.

Eversion—Rotation of the foot outward, hurts like hell; opposite of inversion. Both of them can hurt like heck.

Fat—The reason you're reading this book. One gram gives you nine calories, so you don't need a lot to get a lot. Phat is something different; that means bad to the bone, slick, or bumpin' . . .

Fatigue—Being tired; suck it up and deal with it. You bring it on faster if you don't warm up and cool down.

Flexibility—Range of motion; the result of doing the Sarge's stretches.

Glucose—Sugar in blood. You need this to burn fat, therefore, to create energy. If you have too much of it, though, it is stored—simply stored—and you know what that means to your hips.

HDL—High-density lipoprotein, or "good cholesterol" because it removes excess cholesterol from the body. Also, see "LDL," or low-density lipoprotein. (Remember the saying, "You want the high high and the low, low.")

Heart attack—Read this book and follow it, and you probably won't need to know.

Heat exhaustion—A heat-related illness that is common, because there are lots of jerkies who think they can jog in hot, humid weather without carrying a water bottle and using it. Bad, prolonged sweating takes the fluids right out of you. Next thing you know, you fall over and some Good Samaritan does CPR on you. See CPR.

Heat stroke—Pay attention, boys and girls, this could kill you! A person suffering from heat stroke no longer sweats because the body's heat-regulating system shuts down.

Hips—Ask any woman over thirty.

Hypertension—High blood pressure (140/90 or over). See a doctor, quit your job, get in shape. I'm not kidding.

Hypertrophy—Muscle growth—not number of muscles, smart-ass—size.

Hyperventilation—What happens to your breathing when you don't follow Sarge's four-part breathing technique during your run. Breathing at a fast rate like that can make you dizzy, so slow down.

Hypoglycemia—Low blood sugar. It can happen to a diabetic who is exercising too hard.

Inversion—Rotation of the foot inward, hurts like hell; opposite of eversion.

Isometric contraction—A contraction in which the muscle is working, but not changing in length. When you are really crunching in a crunch, you are doing an isometric contraction with your abs.

Jackass—See jerky.

Jerky—Smart aleck.

Jolly Fat Man's Run—Held every December in Washington, D.C., for members of our fitness program. The purpose of it is to get all our people together to do a fun run.

Ketosis—If you cut carbs from your diet, fast, or starve yourself, this is what will happen. Not only is it an unhealthy condition, your breath smells rank all the time.

Kinesthetic awareness—A sense of position and movement in space; great athletes have a lot of it. If you can pass a drunk driving test, you have some.

Kyphosis—A curve in the upper back that makes you look like the Hunchback of Notre Dame.

Lactic acid (lactate)—A by-product of anaerobic activity.

Lactose—Sugar within milk. Some people have little tolerance to it.

Lame ass—See poopy pants.

Lard ass—Big-butted, slow-moving recruit.

Lateral movement—Movement away from midline of body; opposite of medial.

LDL—Low-density lipid protein; called "bad cholesterol," because it's the kind that clogs your arteries. See HDL.

Ligament—Tissue that connects bone to bone.

Lipid—Fat.

Liver lips—See jerky.

Lordosis—Excessive lumbar curve; swayback.

Maximal heart rate—As fast as your heart can go.

Maximal oxygen consumption (VO2 max)—Maximum aerobic capacity; the maximum amount of oxygen you can consume while you exercise.

Meniscus—Cushioning tissue found within the knee; shock absorber in the knee.

Mesomorph—Thick muscular body like Sarge's.

Metabolism—Chemical reaction of a cell that turns materials into energy.

Muffin-ass—My most endearing term for a recruit.

Muscular endurance—Capacity of a muscle to do something repeatedly that requires strength. (Drop and give me twenty!)

Muscular strength—The maximum amount of force you can put out in a single effort. Remember when that meant one pull-up?

On the line—Be prepared to exercise.

Overuse injury—An injury caused by too much stress, over and over, on one part of the body.

Obesity—A superfat condition; usually refers to men who have more than 25 percent body fat and women who have more than 30 percent.

Passive stretch—See static stretch.

Poopy pants—Sergeant Ahmad's name for a lazy recruit.

Private—Someone new to the program.

Protein—You need it to build and repair tissues in the body. One gram gives you four calories.

Rating of perceived exertion—A scale that helps you figure out how easy or hard an exercise is; it's based totally on how you feel. You might be able to fool the Sarge every once in a while, but you can't fool yourself.

Recover—An order meaning, "Stop exercising."

Relax—See recover.

Report (emphasis on re)—An order meaning, "Tell me what you ate yesterday."

RICE—Rest, Ice, Compression, Elevation; the most common way to treat a musculoskeletal injury.

ROM—Range of motion (stretch and this will never be a problem for you, soldier).

Saturated fat—Fatty acid that carries the maximum number of hydrogen atoms; fat of death; atom bomb. Solid at room temperature and in your blood vessels. Most likely, the source of it had a mother.

Scholiosis—Abnormal curvature of the spine.

Sergeant—Your instructor, the great one who teaches and insults.

Sergeant's Private Moment—That special time before you work out when you read a good magazine in Sergeant's Special Room.

Sergeant's Special Room—It ain't the gym, chisel chest.

Shin splint—Delayed pain commonly found in front of lower leg. Should stop when the activity that is aggravating it is stopped. If not, could be a stress fracture; get out your checkbook and visit the doctor to be sure.

Side stitch—Sharp pain in the side; caused by lack of oxygen flow to respiratory muscles. See diaphragm.

Slacker—A slow-going or do-nothing lazy-ass recruit.

Smoke it—An order that means, "Go to fatigue," no, "Go beyond fatigue."

Spot reduction—A fallacy; a joke, unless you hire a plastic surgeon. You can't get rid of fat in a particular area by exercising, no matter what they tell you on the infomercials.

Sprain—A joint twist that hurts like hell. RICE it. It's usually the result of taking a ligament past its normal length.

Static (passive) stretch—A long duration stretch with no bouncing; you maintain constant tension with the muscle. All the stretches in Boot Camp are static.

Strain—Muscle pull or slight tear.

Strength—Ability to move an object once. In Boot Camp, that object is your body.

Stress fracture—A crack in the outer lining of a bone. Yeoww, Sarge can't help. You must see a doctor; it's time to pay up.

Systolic pressure—Pressure exerted by the blood on the blood vessel walls when the heart contracts. It is the higher number in 120/80. Also, see "diastolic."

Tendinitis—Inflammation of a tendon. You're not bouncing when you stretch, are you?

Tendon—Band of tissue that connects muscle to bone.

Tough guy—One who tries to impress the Sarge. Oh, how many try and so many fail!

Valsalva maneuver—Holding your breath and bearing down. The meatheads in the gym do it all the time when they lift heavy weights. Jacks your blood pressure through the roof; can cause hemorrhoids and strokes. Don't do it when you exercise—ever!

Vein—A blood vessel that carries blood to heart.

Warm-up—Mild exercise before vigorous exercise; designed to prevent injury. Puts perspiration on your forehead.

Wingnut—My coauthor Maryann.

Worthless bag of atrophy—A no-muscle smart aleck; a skinny jackass.

APPENDIX A

BODY COMPOSITION TABLES FOR MALE
AND FEMALE RECRUITS
(Source: ARA Human Factors)

LISTEN UP!

If you do not see your height or circumference values on these charts, just extrapolate from the numbers given.

And remember: These numbers are an approximation.

BODY COMPOSITION TABLE—MALES

waist minus neck	Height										
	62	62.5	63	63.5	64	64.5	65	65.5	66	66.5	67
11	2	1	1	1	1	1	-	-	-	-	-
11.5	3	3	3	2	2	2	2	2	1	1	1
12	5	4	4	4	4	3	3	3	3	3	2
12.5	6	6	6	5	5	5	5	4	4	4	4
13	7	7	7	7	6	6	6	6	6	5	5
13.5	9	8	8	8	8	8	7	7	7	7	6
14	10	10	10	9	9	9	9	8	8	8	8
14.4	11	11	11	11	10	10	10	10	9	9	9
15	12	12	12	12	11	11	11	11	11	10	10
15.5	14	13	13	13	12	12	12	12	12	12	11
16	15	15	14	14	13	14	13	13	13	13	12
16.5	16	16	15	15	14	15	14	14	14	14	14
17	17	17	16	16	15	16	16	15	15	15	15
17.5	18	18	18	17	16	17	17	16	16	16	16
18	18	19	19	18	17	18	18	17	17	17	17
18.5	20	20	20	19	18	19	19	18	18	18	18
19	21	21	21	20	19	20	20	19	19	19	19
19.5	22	22	22	21	20	21	21	20	20	20	20
20	23	23	22	22	21	22	22	21	21	21	21
20.5	24	24	23	23	22	23	22	22	22	22	22
21	25	25	24	24	23	24	23	23	23	23	22
21.5	26	25	25	25	24	24	24	24	24	24	23
22	27	26	26	26	25	25	25	25	25	24	24
22.5	27	27	27	27	26	26	26	26	25	25	25
23	28	28	28	28	26	27	27	27	26	26	26
23.5	29	29	29	28	27	28	28	27	27	27	27
24	30	30	29	29	28	29	28	28	28	28	27
24.5	31	30	30	30	29	29	29	29	29	29	28
25	31	31	31	31	30	30	30	30	29	29	29
25.5	32	32	32	31	31	31	31	31	30	30	30
26	33	33	32	32	32	32	32	31	31	31	31
26.5	34	33	33	33	33	32	32	32	32	32	31
27	34	34	34	34	33	33	33	33	32	32	32
27.5	35	35	35	34	34	34	34	33	33	33	33
28	36	36	35	35	35	35	34	34	34	34	33
28.5	37	36	36	36	36	35	35	35	34	34	34
29	37	37	37	37	36	36	36	36	35	35	35
29.5	38	37	37	37	37	37	36	36	36	36	35
30	39	38	38	38	38	37	37	37	37	36	36
30.5	39	39	39	39	38	38	38	38	37	37	37
31	40	40	39	39	39	39	38	38	38	38	37
31.5				40	40	39	39	39	39	38	38
32						40	40	39	39	39	39
32.5									40	40	39
33											40
33.5											
34											
34.5					If you belong here, see your doctor NOW!						
35											

BODY COMPOSITION TABLE—MALES

waist minus neck	Height										
	67.5	68	68.5	69	69.5	70	70.5	71	71.5	72	72.5
11.5	1	1	-	-	-	-	-	-	-	-	-
12	2	2	2	2	1	1	1	1	1	-	-
12.5	4	3	3	3	3	3	2	2	2	2	2
13	5	5	5	4	4	4	4	4	3	3	3
13.5	6	6	6	6	5	5	5	5	5	4	4
14	8	7	7	7	7	7	6	6	6	6	6
14.5	9	9	8	8	8	8	8	7	7	7	7
15	10	10	10	9	9	9	9	9	8	8	8
15.5	11	11	11	11	10	10	10	10	9	9	9
16	12	12	12	12	11	11	11	11	11	10	10
16.5	13	13	13	13	13	12	12	12	12	12	11
17	14	14	14	14	14	13	13	13	13	13	12
17.5	16	15	15	15	15	14	14	14	14	14	13
18	17	16	16	16	16	15	15	15	15	15	14
18.5	18	17	17	17	17	16	16	16	16	16	15
19	19	18	18	18	18	17	17	17	17	17	16
19.5	19	19	19	19	19	18	18	18	18	18	17
20	20	20	20	20	20	19	19	19	19	18	18
20.5	21	21	21	21	20	20	20	20	20	19	19
21	22	22	22	22	21	21	21	21	20	20	20
21.5	23	23	23	22	22	22	22	22	21	21	21
22	24	24	24	23	23	23	23	22	22	22	22
22.5	25	25	24	24	24	24	23	23	23	23	23
23	26	25	25	25	25	25	24	24	24	24	23
23.5	26	26	26	26	26	25	25	25	25	24	24
24	27	27	27	27	26	26	26	26	25	25	25
24.5	28	28	28	27	27	27	27	26	26	26	26
25	29	29	28	28	28	28	27	27	27	27	27
25.5	30	29	29	29	29	28	28	28	28	28	27
26	30	30	30	30	29	29	29	29	29	28	28
26.5	31	31	31	30	30	30	30	29	29	29	29
27	32	32	31	31	31	31	30	30	30	30	30
27.5	33	32	32	32	32	31	31	31	31	30	30
28	33	33	33	33	32	32	32	32	31	31	31
28.5	34	34	33	33	33	33	33	32	32	32	32
29	35	34	34	34	34	33	33	33	33	33	32
29.5	35	35	35	35	34	34	34	34	33	33	33
30	36	36	35	35	35	35	35	34	34	34	34
30.5	37	36	36	36	36	35	35	35	35	35	34
31	37	37	37	37	36	36	36	36	35	35	35
31.5	38	38	37	37	37	37	36	36	36	36	36
32	38	38	38	38	38	37	37	37	37	36	36
32.5	39	39	39	38	38	38	38	37	37	37	37
33	40	39	39	39	39	39	38	38	38	38	37
33.5			40	40	39	39	39	39	38	38	38
34					40	40	39	39	39	39	39
34.5								40	40	39	39
35										40	40
35.5											

BODY COMPOSITION TABLE—MALES

waist minus neck	Height										
	73	73.5	74	74.5	75	75.5	76	76.5	77	77.5	78
13	3	3	-	-	-	-	-	-	-	-	-
13.5	4	4	4	4	3	3	3	3	3	2	2
14	5	5	5	5	5	4	4	4	4	4	3
14.5	7	6	6	6	6	6	5	5	5	5	5
15	8	8	7	7	7	7	7	6	6	6	6
15.5	9	9	9	8	8	8	8	8	7	7	7
16	10	10	10	9	9	9	9	9	8	8	8
16.5	11	11	11	11	10	10	10	10	10	9	9
17	12	12	12	12	11	11	11	11	11	10	10
17.5	13	13	13	13	12	12	12	12	12	11	11
18	14	14	14	14	13	13	13	13	13	12	12
18.5	15	15	15	15	14	14	14	14	14	13	13
19	16	16	16	16	15	15	15	15	15	14	14
19.5	17	17	17	17	16	16	16	16	16	15	15
20	18	18	18	17	17	17	17	17	16	16	16
20.5	19	19	19	18	18	18	18	18	17	17	17
21	20	20	19	19	19	19	19	18	18	18	18
21.5	21	21	20	20	20	20	20	19	19	19	19
22	22	21	21	21	21	21	20	20	20	20	20
22.5	22	22	22	22	22	21	21	21	21	21	20
23	23	23	23	23	22	22	22	22	22	21	21
23.5	24	24	24	23	23	23	23	23	22	22	22
24	25	25	24	24	24	24	24	23	23	23	23
24.5	26	25	25	25	25	25	24	24	24	24	24
25	26	26	26	26	26	25	25	25	25	25	24
25.5	27	27	27	27	26	26	26	26	26	25	25
26	28	28	27	27	27	27	27	26	26	26	26
26.5	29	28	28	28	28	28	27	27	27	27	27
27	29	29	29	29	28	28	28	28	28	27	27
27.5	30	30	30	29	29	29	29	29	28	28	28
28	31	31	30	30	30	30	29	29	29	29	29
28.5	31	31	31	31	31	30	30	30	30	30	29
29	32	32	32	31	31	31	31	31	30	30	30
29.5	33	33	32	32	32	32	31	31	31	31	31
30	33	33	33	33	33	32	32	32	32	32	31
30.5	34	34	34	33	33	33	33	33	32	32	32
31	35	34	34	34	34	34	33	33	33	33	33
31.5	35	35	35	35	34	34	34	34	34	33	33
32	36	36	36	35	35	35	35	34	34	34	34
32.5	37	36	36	36	36	35	35	35	35	35	35
33	37	37	37	37	36	36	36	36	35	35	35
33.5	38	38	37	37	37	37	36	36	36	36	36
34	38	38	38	38	37	37	37	37	37	36	36
34.5	39	39	39	38	38	38	38	37	37	37	37
35	40	39	39	39	39	38	38	38	38	38	37
35.5					39	39	39	39	38	38	38
36					40	40	39	39	39	39	39
36.5							40	40	39	39	39
37										40	40

BODY COMPOSITION TABLE—FEMALES

waist plus hip minus neck	Height 60	60.5	61	61.5	62	62.5	63	63.5	64	64.5	65
35.5	1	1									
36	2	2	1	1	1						
36.5	3	3	2	2	2	1	1	1			
37	4	4	3	3	3	2	2	2	1	1	1
37.5	5	5	4	4	4	3	3	3	2	2	2
38	6	6	5	5	5	4	4	3	3	3	2
38.5	7	7	6	6	5	5	5	4	4	4	3
39	8	7	7	7	6	6	6	5	5	5	4
39.5	9	8	8	8	7	7	7	6	6	6	5
40	10	9	9	8	8	8	7	7	7	6	6
40.5	10	10	10	9	9	9	8	8	8	7	7
41	11	11	11	10	10	10	9	9	8	8	8
41.5	12	12	11	11	11	10	10	10	9	9	9
42	13	13	12	12	12	11	11	10	10	10	9
42.5	14	13	13	13	12	12	12	11	11	11	10
43	15	14	14	14	13	13	12	12	12	11	11
43.5	15	15	15	14	14	14	13	13	13	12	12
44	16	16	16	15	15	14	14	14	13	13	13
44.5	17	17	16	16	16	15	15	15	14	14	14
45	18	17	17	17	16	16	16	15	15	15	14
45.5	19	18	18	18	17	17	16	16	16	15	15
46	19	19	19	18	18	18	17	17	17	16	16
46.5	20	20	19	19	19	18	18	18	17	17	16
47	21	20	20	20	19	19	19	18	18	18	17
47.5	22	21	21	21	20	20	19	19	19	18	18
48	22	22	22	22	21	21	20	20	20	19	19
48.5	23	23	22	22	22	21	21	21	20	20	20
49	24	23	23	23	22	22	22	21	21	21	20
49.5	24	24	24	23	23	23	22	22	22	21	21
50	25	25	24	24	24	23	23	23	22	22	22
50.5	26	26	25	25	24	24	24	23	23	23	22
51	27	26	26	25	25	25	24	24	24	23	23
51.5	27	27	27	26	26	25	25	25	24	24	24
52	28	28	27	27	27	26	26	25	25	25	24
52.5	29	28	28	28	27	27	26	26	26	25	25
53	29	29	29	28	28	27	27	27	26	26	26
53.5	30	30	29	29	28	28	28	27	27	27	27
54	31	30	30	30	29	29	28	28	28	27	27
54.5	31	31	31	30	30	29	29	29	28	28	28
55	32	32	31	31	30	30	30	29	29	29	28
55.5	33	32	32	31	31	31	30	30	30	29	29
56	33	33	32	32	32	31	31	30	30	30	30
56.6	34	33	33	33	32	32	32	31	31	31	30
57	34	34	34	33	33	33	32	32	32	31	31
57.5	35	35	34	34	34	33	33	32	32	32	31
58	36	35	35	35	34	34	33	33	33	32	32
58.5	36	36	35	35	35	34	34	34	33	33	33
59	37	36	36	36	35	35	35	34	34	34	33
59.5	37	37	37	36	36	36	35	35	35	34	34
60	38	38	37	37	37	37	36	35	35	35	34

BODY COMPOSITION TABLE—FEMALES

waist plus hip minus neck	Height										
	65.5	66	66.5		67	67.5	68	68.5	69	69.5	70
37											
37.5	1	1	1								
38	2	2	1		1	1					
38.5	3	3	2		2	2	1	1	1	1	
39	4	4	3		3	3	2	2	2	2	
39.5	5	5	4		4	4	3	3	3	3	1
40	6	5	5		5	4	4	4	3	4	2
40.5	7	6	6		6	5	5	5	4	5	3
41	7	7	7		6	6	6	5	5	5	4
41.5	8	8	8		7	7	7	6	6	6	5
42	9	9	8		8	8	8	7	7	7	6
42.5	10	10	9		9	9	8	8	8	8	7
43	11	10	10		10	9	9	9	9	9	8
43.5	12	11	11		11	10	10	10	9	9	9
44	12	12	12		11	11	11	10	10	10	9
44.5	13	13	13		12	12	12	11	11	11	9
45	14	14	13		13	13	12	12	12	12	10
45.5	15	14	14		14	13	13	13	12	13	11
46	16	15	15		15	14	14	14	13	13	12
46.5	16	16	16		15	15	15	14	14	14	13
47	17	17	16		16	16	15	15	15	15	13
47.5	18	17	17		17	16	16	16	15	16	14
48	18	18	18		18	17	17	17	16	16	15
48.5	19	19	19		18	18	18	17	17	17	16
49	20	20	19		19	19	18	18	18	18	16
49.5	21	20	20		20	19	19	19	18	18	17
50	21	21	21		20	20	20	19	19	19	18
50.5	22	22	21		21	21	20	20	20	20	18
51	23	22	22		22	21	21	21	20	20	19
51.5	23	23	23		22	22	22	21	21	21	20
52	24	24	23		23	23	22	22	22	22	21
52.5	25	24	24		24	23	23	23	22	23	21
53	25	25	25		24	24	24	23	23	23	22
53.5	26	26	25		25	25	24	24	24	24	23
54	27	26	26		26	25	25	25	24	24	23
54.5	27	27	27		26	26	26	25	25	25	24
55	28	28	27		27	27	26	26	26	26	24
55.5	29	28	28		28	27	27	27	26	26	25
56	29	29	29		28	28	28	27	27	27	26
56.5	30	30	29		29	29	28	28	28	28	26
57	31	30	30		30	29	29	29	28	28	27
57.5	31	31	30		30	30	30	29	29	29	28
58	32	31	31		31	30	30	30	29	29	28
58.5	32	32	32		31	31	31	30	30	30	29
59	33	33	33		32	32	31	31	31	30	30
59.5	34	34	33		33	33	32	32	31	31	31
60	35	34	34		34	33	32	32	32	32	31
60.5	36	35	35		34	34	33	33	32	32	32
61	36	36	35		35	35	34	33	33	33	32

APPENDIX B

OXYGEN CONSUMPTION FORMULA

Welcome to the oxygen consumption formula, math wiz! This calculation will give you a better sense of your cardiorespiratory fitness than the heart rate number alone, but you have to think. I never said exercise was for dummies!

To do this, you not only have to record your *heart rate* after you finish the mile walk, but also the *time* it took you to walk the mile.

By the way, you don't need to know what the numbers in this formula mean. If you must know, call somebody who has a Ph.D.

MEN

Oxygen consumption = 139.168 − (0.3888 × age) − (0.077 × weight) − (3.265 × mile walk time) − (0.156 × exercise heart rate)

WOMEN

Same formula, but subtract everything from 132.85 instead of 139.168.

EXAMPLE

Mel is forty years old, he weighs 220 pounds, it took him twenty minutes to walk a mile, and his heart was going 120 beats per minute after the walk.

$$
\begin{array}{ll}
139.168 & \\
\underline{-\ \ 15.52} & \text{(That's } 0.388 \times \text{forty years old.)} \\
123.648 & \\
\underline{-\ \ 16.94} & \text{(That's } 0.077 \times 220 \text{ pounds.)} \\
106.708 & \\
\underline{-\ \ 65.30} & \text{(That's } 3.265 \times \text{twenty minutes.)} \\
41.408 & \\
\underline{-\ \ 18.72} & \text{(That's } 0.156 \times 120 \text{ beats per minute.)} \\
=\ 22.688 = \text{Oxygen consumption} &
\end{array}
$$

Remember, if Mel is Melanie, everything is subtracted from 132.85.

When you get your "oxygen consumption" number, check the grid below to see where you want to be based on age. As you can see, Mel needs to kick himself in the butt. What would put him in the "standard" area? If he dumped about twenty pounds of fat and was able to do the walk in seventeen minutes, he'd be in a good range. That's no problem for anybody in MY program!

AEROBIC FITNESS STANDARDS FOR HEALTH[1]

Age Group	Men (O_2 Consumption)	Women (O_2 Consumption)
<45	36	32
50	34	31
55	32	29
60	31	28
>65	30	27

If you don't like where you stand—and you probably won't—get excited, not discouraged. Boot Camp is your chance to change these numbers starting NOW.

[1] Baumgartner, T.A., and A.S. Jackson, *Measurement for Evaluation*, Madison, Brown & Benchmark (1995).

APPENDIX C

NORMS FOR TRUNK FLEXIBILITY TEST (MEN)

| Flexibility | Age (years) | | | | | |
	18–25	26–35	36–45	46–55	56–65	65+
Excellent	>20	>20	>19	>19	>17	>17
Good	18–20	18–19	17–19	16–17	14–17	13–16
Above average	17–18	16–17	15–17	14–15	12–14	11–13
Average	15–16	15–16	13–15	12–13	10–12	9–11
Below average	13–14	12–14	11–13	10–11	8–10	8–9
Poor	10–12	10–12	9–11	7–9	5–8	5–7
Very poor	<10	<10	<8	<7	<5	<5

NORMS FOR TRUNK FLEXIBILITY TEST (WOMEN)

| Flexibility | Age (years) | | | | | |
	18–25	26–35	36–45	46–55	56–65	65+
Excellent	>24	>23	>22	>21	>20	>20
Good	21–23	20–22	19–21	18–20	18–19	18–19
Above average	20–21	19–20	17–19	17–18	16–17	16–17
Average	18–19	18	16–17	15–16	15	14–15
Below average	17–18	16–17	14–15	14–15	13–14	12–13
Poor	14–16	14–15	11–13	11–13	10–12	9–11
Very poor	<13	<13	<10	<10	<9	<8

These charts were reprinted from *Y's Way to Physical Fitness*, 3rd Edition (1989), only with permission of the YMCA of the USA, 101 N. Wacker Drive, Chicago, IL 60606.

APPENDIX D

HEALTH, FITNESS AND NUTRITION

www.sarge.com

Our official Web site lets you know what Sarge does with his time, other than write books. To ask questions about Boot Camp or seek help with your fitness program, send E-mail. If you're desperate, E-mail *me* at sarge@sarge.com.

www.shapeup.org

Shape Up America! Campaign, established by Dr. C. Everett Koop, the former surgeon general of the United States, is designed to educate the public on the importance of increased physical activity and the achievement and maintenance of a healthy body weight. This site supports that mission.

www.afpafitness.com

You can find a wealth of information on nutrition, exercise, and training in the "health facts articles" section of the American Fitness Professionals and Associates site.

rampages.onramp.net/~chaz/

The primary purpose of the Internet's Fitness Resource is the dissemination of information on exercise and nutrition. It contains links to fitness-related sites.

www.teamoregon.com/~teamore/ publications/mags.html

This is the portion of Team Oregon's site that provides links to online running, walking, and fitness publications, as well as sources of fitness publications in print.

NUTRITION

navigator.tufts.edu

"A rating guide to nutrition Web sites," this site is produced by the Center on Nutrition Communication, School of Nutrition Science and Policy of Tufts University and contains helpful links and information, including "health facts articles."

www.mealsforyou.com

At this site, you can find recipes and meals described in terms of preparation time, cooking time, and calories, as well as fat, cholesterol, and sodium content.

INDEX